The Balanced Path

Unlock the Secret to a Healthier, Happier
Life with Hara Hachi Bu

JOSEPH KASA~VUBU

Table of Content

Introduction to Hara Hachi Bu

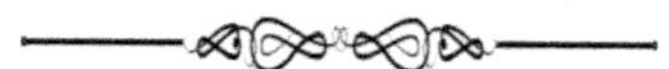

What if the secret to a longer and healthier life could be summed up in just three words? Imagine a life where each meal leaves you feeling lighter, more energized, and brimming with the vitality of someone years younger. Could our journey toward this vibrant existence be hidden in an ancient practice that's as simple as it is profound? Welcome to the world of Hara Hachi Bu—an age-old wisdom revered by the centenarians of Okinawa, renowned for their remarkable longevity and zest for life. This simple concept could hold the key to transforming not just how we eat but also how we live.

Picture yourself in the lush and serene landscapes of Okinawa, where life seems to flow gently, and each meal is more than just sustenance. Food embodies a way of life amongst the whispering winds and rolling green hills. Individuals have thrived in this idyllic setting for centuries, revealing secrets to a long and fulfilling life. Hara Hachi Bu is central to their thriving existence, a mindful practice that elevates meals to treasured moments of connection and balance. In Okinawa, moderation isn't just advised—it's celebrated. Through meals that delight the senses without overwhelming them, this philosophy speaks of harmony and health.

Imagine tapping into this profound knowledge from your dining room table. The benefits of adopting Hara Hachi Bu extend far beyond eating. Those who embrace this lifestyle choice often have renewed mental clarity and emotional well-being. Lowered risk of chronic diseases and a palpable boost in overall happiness become part of their everyday reality. It's an approach that fosters a deeper appreciation for food, encouraging better physical health and nurturing emotional and social well-being.

But why now? Why has this ancient practice never been more relevant than in today's fast-paced world? In our society, where convenience frequently precedes mindfulness, the call to adopt Hara Hachi Bu has gained urgency. Are you tired of feeling sluggish after meals or struggling under immense pressure to consume, do, and be more? The modern-day challenges of overeating and unhealthy lifestyle choices are undeniable. Yet, within these challenges lies the opportunity for profound transformation. The time to reconsider our habits and make meaningful changes is here, standing at the threshold of our current lifestyles, inviting us to evolve.

This book isn't just about food; it's a guide—a supportive companion on your journey towards enhanced well-being. As you delve into the pages ahead, you'll uncover rich traditions and practical strategies deeply rooted in Okinawan culture. These pages empower you to take charge of your health, one mindful meal at a time, by understanding and integrating Hara Hachi Bu's principles. We'll navigate this journey together, exploring the profound wisdom nurtured over generations in Okinawa—a wisdom that's not only applicable but crucial for contemporary living.

Through stories, insights, and step-by-step guidance, this book invites you to rethink your relationship with food and embrace a lifestyle that promises longevity and fulfillment. Imagine a life overflowing with energy, joy, and good health—a life where every bite contributes to a fuller existence. It begins with three simple words and a commitment to pursue a more mindful and rewarding path.

Let's embark on this transformative journey, honoring the rhythms of nature and the wisdom of those who've walked before us. Join us in redefining what it means to live well and thrive, using the power of mindful eating to unlock a future brimming with possibilities.

Your future self will thank you as each mindful decision brings you closer to a life enriched with purpose, joy, and years of cherished moments.

Welcome to the beginning of your journey toward a longer, healthier, and more remarkable life. Let the adventure begin.

"Three grand essentials to happiness in this life are
something to do,
something to love and
something to hope for."
Addison

Chapter 1

The Essence
of Hara Hachi Bu

Hara Hachi Bu is a centuries-old practice originating from Okinawa, an island known for its bountiful natural beauty and the remarkable longevity of its people. It offers more than just dietary advice; it embodies a holistic lifestyle deeply ingrained in cultural and historical roots. This principle gently nudges us to stop eating when we feel 80% full, guiding us toward moderation without deprivation. The concept is deceptively simple yet profound in its impact on health and well-being, offering a testament to how tradition and modern insight can mesh seamlessly to foster vitality.

In this chapter, readers will journey through the fascinating origins of Hara Hachi Bu within Okinawan culture, exploring how these dietary habits emerged from a tapestry of history, geography, and community values. The narrative reveals how Okinawans have crafted an existence that harmonizes with their environment, celebrating food as nourishment and cultural expression.

From understanding the influence of the island's subtropical climate and trade routes to examining the enduring traditions shaped by communal resilience and resourcefulness, readers will discover the intricate connections that lead to a healthier, balanced way of life. Through this exploration, a deeper appreciation will emerge of how Hara Hachi Bu transcends mere nutritional guidance to become a meaningful part of a lifestyle that promises longevity and joy.

Historical Background of Okinawa's Dietary Habits

Okinawa, a beautiful archipelago in Japan, is home to some of the longest-living people on Earth, and much of this longevity is credited to their unique dietary practices. Nestled between China, Taiwan, and the main Japanese islands, Okinawa's geography has played a pivotal role in shaping its cuisine. The climate is subtropical, ideal for growing various fruits and vegetables that contribute to a diet rich in nutrients yet low in calories. Historically, this region has been a melting pot of cultures due to trade routes and various territorial influences, resulting in a diverse culinary tradition that blends elements from Chinese, Southeast Asian, and Japanese cuisines.

Nevertheless, it's not only geography and history that have left a mark on Okinawan dietary habits; cultural traditions also play a critical role. Cuisine here is more than just sustenance—it embodies community values and historical resilience. Take, for example, the tradition of sharing food among families and neighbors, infusing each meal with a sense of community and moderation. This concept will eventually manifest into the practice known as Hara Hachi Bu, but first, it's essential to understand the roots of these dietary customs.

Examining the traditional Okinawan diet reveals that it emphasizes low-calorie density foods packed with nutrients. Staples include sweet potatoes, which replaced rice after being introduced from the Americas, while seafood provides a lean source of protein. Locally grown vegetables such as Goya (bitter melon), daikon radish, and leafy greens are dietary mainstays, along with tofu and whole grains. These foods nourish the body with essential vitamins and minerals and contribute to feeling full without excessive calorie intake.

This approach to eating fosters both satiety and health, setting a foundation for understanding Hara Hachi Bu—a principle advocating eating until one is 80% full. In essence, the food culture promotes quality over quantity, encouraging individuals to delight in the flavors and textures of their meals while maintaining a balanced intake.

World War II profoundly changed Okinawa's way of life, significantly impacting food consumption patterns. The war led to scarcity and hardship, urging people to make do with limited resources. Resourcefulness became a way of life, influencing today's attitudes toward food. Communities had to rely heavily on locally available produce and collaborate closely, reinforcing bonds through shared adversity. Even post-war, this emphasis on resourcefulness continued, becoming emblematic of Okinawan perseverance and adaptability.

The scarcity faced during WWII fostered a deep appreciation for food, transforming mealtime into a meaningful ritual where nothing went to waste, and every meal was a testament to survival. This era ingrained the value of mindfulness around consumption, further embedding the principles of resourcefulness and gratitude—a reflection of the communal spirit that defines Okinawan culture.

In more modern times, the evolution of mindful eating has made its mark on these communal practices, promoting moderation, enjoyment, and strong social ties. Eating in Okinawa is rarely rushed; meals are often leisurely filled with conversation and laughter. This unhurried style encourages savoring each bite, creating opportunities to experience the deliciousness and the emotional nourishment of eating together.

Mindful eating practices encourage moderation by fostering awareness of hunger cues and fullness signals. Okinawans naturally integrate these practices into their routines, reflecting their broader cultural commitment to living harmoniously with nature and honoring family traditions. Communal dining experiences emphasize connections between people, reinforcing bonds and providing a sense of belonging that contributes positively to mental well-being.

As Okinawa continues to embrace these age-old practices while adapting to modern challenges, it showcases how a culture deeply rooted in history, geography, and community can yield powerful insights into healthy living. Understanding the origins and evolution of dietary practices in Okinawa sets the stage for appreciating Hara Hachi Bu's philosophy. This principle is not solely about eating less but about cultivating an intentional relationship with food that balances nutritional intake with cultural significance and personal well-being.

Vital Elements of Mindful Eating Practices

The principles of mindful eating are at the heart of the Hara Hachi Bu philosophy, originating in Okinawan culture. These principles guide individuals to engage with food more thoughtfully and meaningfully. The practice begins with awareness—tuning into the body's natural hunger and fullness signals. In modern life, becoming disconnected from these signals is easy, often leading to mindless eating habits. However, paying attention when you're genuinely hungry or comfortably full encourages a healthier relationship with food. This connection helps dissociate food from guilt or emotional eating, fostering a sense of balance.

Imagine being at a table with a colorful array of foods before you. Rather than diving in without thought, take a moment to appreciate the visual appeal, the aroma wafting up, signaling your anticipation. This is where savoring each bite comes into play. Eating slowly and deliberately allows for sensory engagement, enhancing satisfaction even with smaller meal portions. By focusing on taste, texture, and aroma, you can derive greater pleasure from your meals and naturally avoid overeating. When each mouthful is an experience, it becomes easier to recognize when enough is enough.

Beyond individual practices, the cultural rituals surrounding dining also contribute substantially to mindful eating. In many cultures, communal dining is not just about consuming food; it's about sharing experiences, stories, and gratitude. On the islands of Okinawa, shared meals are a ritual—a time to express thankfulness not just for the food but for the company and the moment itself. Such practices encourage an appreciation for each meal, transforming dining into an event rather than a routine.

In the context of Hara Hachi Bu, portion control is another essential strategy. While the concept might evoke images of restriction, it's more about understanding what your body needs. With a mindful approach, portion control becomes less about eating less and more about eating smarter. It's about balance—ensuring that what goes on your plate supports your overall well-being. Simple strategies like using smaller plates or pre-plating meals help regulate intake gently but effectively.

Guidelines recommended for practicing mindful portion control emphasize starting with small portions and then assessing whether you're still hungry before reaching for more. This method respects the body's signals and avoids overindulgence. It's a practical way to align eating with thoughtful intention while respecting one's nutritional requirements.

Awareness of these eating habits can pave the path for a healthier lifestyle. It encourages reflection on how much and why we eat. Developing this mindfulness takes practice. Begin by setting aside dedicated mealtimes without distractions, such as phones or televisions, allowing focus solely on the meal. Over time, you'll find yourself making choices aligned with actual needs rather than impulses driven by stress or convenience.

The beauty of savoring lies in its simplicity. Mindful eating doesn't require exotic ingredients or complex recipes, just the commitment to be present with each meal. As you commence this journey, slow down, breathe between bites, and allow each flavor to unfold fully. You'll discover that satisfaction increases exponentially when meals aren't rushed but relished.

Cultural rituals can further enrich this practice. Reflect on meals shared with loved ones—the laughter, the stories told over steaming bowls of soup, or during a leisurely Sunday breakfast. Such experiences underscore the importance of dining as a collective, reflective act. Taking moments to be thankful, whether through a silent note of gratitude or words shared aloud, enhances the experience, adding depth to simple acts of nourishment.

Meanwhile, portion control becomes part of daily life as a sustainable habit rather than a fleeting diet trend. Serving sensible amounts initially, possibly inspired by traditional serving sizes rooted in seasonality and availability, promotes enduring health benefits. Adjustments to portioning reflect an understanding of personal energy needs that change over time, influenced by activity levels, age, and health status.

Integrating these principles fosters a dynamic interaction with eating. It encourages viewing meals as opportunities to connect with one's self and community, nourishing both body and spirit. As individuals embrace Hara Hachi Bu, they cultivate harmony with food, learning to trust in their instincts and wisdom regarding consumption.

Connection Between Hara Hachi Bu and Longevity

Hara Hachi Bu, a simple yet profound practice deeply rooted in Okinawan culture, illuminates a path to health and longevity through mindful eating. At its heart, this philosophy encourages stopping eating when one is 80% full, effectively fostering a habit of low caloric intake. Recent studies have highlighted the correlation between this practice and longer life expectancy in Okinawa, famously home to some of the world's oldest and healthiest people.

The science backing this approach is robust. Consuming fewer calories can significantly decrease the risk of chronic diseases such as diabetes, heart disease, and obesity—all conditions that are far less prevalent among Okinawans compared to their Western counterparts. By naturally regulating calorie intake through Hara Hachi Bu, individuals reduce the overall strain on their bodies, promoting longevity.

Physiologically, this practice offers several benefits. Eating less helps improve metabolic health by maintaining steady blood sugar levels and reducing the likelihood of insulin resistance. Furthermore, it reduces inflammation—a root cause of many chronic diseases—helping the body's systems run more smoothly. Cellular health also thrives under these conditions; reduced calorie consumption promotes autophagy, a process where cells clean out damaged components, thus protecting against illnesses and aging.

The psychological advantages of Hara Hachi Bu are equally compelling. Practicing this form of mindful eating nurtures a healthy relationship with food. Instead of seeing meals as opportunities for indulgence, those embracing Hara Hachi Bu view eating as a chance to nourish their bodies respectfully. This mindset shift can reduce emotional eating and anxiety around food choices, leading to greater emotional resilience.

Additionally, social factors in Okinawa amplify the effects of Hara Hachi Bu. The island's community-oriented lifestyle plays a crucial role in holistic well-being. Meals are often shared experiences steeped in tradition and connection, reinforcing feelings of belonging and happiness. This communal aspect of dining brings joy and encourages moderation, reflecting the respect for food embedded in Okinawan culture.

Moreover, an active lifestyle complements this dietary practice. Okinawans maintain physical activity through formal exercise, which is embedded into daily routines. Gardening, walking, and engaging in traditional dance are everyday activities that keep them moving. Such regular activity supports cardiovascular health, muscle strength, and mental clarity, extending their years and quality of life.

Together, these elements create a synergistic effect contributing to the notable longevity observed in Okinawa. Hara Hachi Bu is more than just a guideline; it's a lifestyle choice intertwined with cultural identity and community values. It teaches us a vital lesson: by listening to our bodies and respecting the natural signals they send, we can lead healthier, more fulfilled lives.

Understanding Hara Hachi Bu's broader impacts involves recognizing its role in constructing a framework for sustainable health practices. It reminds us that small changes, like adjusting how much we eat, can significantly influence long-term health outcomes. This practice illustrates the power of moderation and underscores the importance of integrating cultural wisdom with scientific insights.

Incorporating such strategies into one's life may seem challenging initially, especially in cultures accustomed to abundance and indulgence. However, adopting Hara Hachi Bu requires gradual shifts rather than dramatic overhauls. By paying closer attention to hunger cues or savoring each bite, individuals can develop a more intuitive understanding of their needs, reminiscent of the principles advocated by this Okinawan custom.

Concluding Thoughts

At the heart of Okinawan culture lies the philosophy of Hara Hachi Bu, a practice that encourages stopping eating when one is 80% full. This chapter explored how this simple yet profound idea promotes health and longevity, rooted in generations-old traditions. It's remarkable how geography, history, and cultural values blend and thrive on this Japanese island, fostering a mindful relationship with food. Instilling respect for nature's bounty and emphasizing community ties through shared meals, Okinawans have crafted a unique dining approach that nurtures physical and emotional well-being.

By embracing these practices, Okinawans offer a glimpse into a lifestyle where food is more than sustenance—an art form woven with gratitude, mindfulness, and connection. The natural alignment with portion control and camaraderie around the table underscores the significance of enjoying meals without haste or excess. As we learn from their experiences, it becomes evident that adopting such mindful eating habits can contribute to a healthier, more balanced life. It's about savoring moments, cherishing connections, and respecting our bodies, reminding us that proper nourishment feeds both body and spirit.

Be grateful for what you already have while you pursue your goals. If you aren't grateful for what you already have, what makes you think you would be happy with more." Roy T. Bennett

Chapter 2

Understanding Mindful Eating

Mindful eating is about tuning in to your body's hunger signals and distinguishing them from mere cravings. It involves embracing awareness and being present with each bite, which can transform how we perceive food and our relationship with it. How often do we eat without even thinking, guided by emotions, or simply because food is there? The concept of mindful eating invites us to pause and reflect, creating a harmonious connection between our mind, body, and meals. This chapter delves into how discerning genuine hunger and emotional triggers can guide us toward healthier eating habits.

Throughout this exploring journey, you'll discover practical insights on differentiating true hunger from cravings, including recognizing physical cues such as a growling stomach versus emotional prompts like stress-driven snacking. We will also uncover the importance of situational influences on our eating patterns. By examining these aspects, the chapter emphasizes making conscious, balanced choices that align with your body's needs. Prepare to engage with techniques that integrate mindfulness into daily meals, learn to enjoy food for its own sake, and cultivate moderation. This practice satisfies and nurtures a lifestyle where physical well-being meets emotional fulfillment.

Distinguishing Hunger from Cravings

Differentiating between genuine hunger and emotional or situational cravings is at the heart of mindful eating. This distinction is crucial in developing healthier eating habits and achieving balance. Let's begin by exploring what genuine physiological hunger feels like. Unlike emotional cravings, physiological hunger is presented through physical sensations such as a growling stomach, feelings of emptiness, or low energy levels. These are signals from the body that it needs nourishment to function optimally. Recognizing these signals allows us to choose nutritious foods that fulfill our body's requirements.

On the other hand, we often find ourselves reaching for food not because we are genuinely hungry but due to emotional triggers. Stress, boredom, sadness, or even celebration can lead to eating when our bodies aren't genuinely asking for it. Imagine a stressful day at work where you instinctively grab a bag of chips not out of hunger but because it provides comfort. Identifying and understanding how these emotional cues affect our eating patterns is essential. Doing so allows us to explore alternative coping mechanisms that do not involve food. Walking, meditating, or engaging in a hobby can effectively manage emotions without eating.

Situations also play a significant role in influencing our eating behavior. Think about social gatherings with abundant food or television evenings and endless snacking. Such external cues often prompt us to eat more than necessary. Recognizing these situational cues can empower us to exercise control over our eating habits. For example, you can focus on the company and conversations during social events rather than mindlessly grazing. Awareness of these settings helps us make more conscious choices about when and what to eat.

Practical exercises can be helpful tools for weaving mindfulness into our daily lives. Reflection before eating is one way to cultivate this habit. Before reaching for food, pause and ask yourself: Am I physically hungry or eating because of an emotion or situation? Taking a moment to assess your true motivation can lead to more mindful decisions. Moreover, keeping a food journal can aid in recognizing patterns related to hunger and cravings, providing insights into how various factors influence your eating behavior.

In addition, practicing mindful breathing can become a helpful pre-meal ritual. Spend a few moments focusing on your breath to center yourself and create a sense of calm. This practice reduces stress-induced eating and enhances your awareness of physiological hunger cues. Over time, these small yet powerful practices reinforce eating mindfully, fostering a deeper connection with your body's needs.

A guideline to distinguish hunger from cravings can be particularly beneficial here. Start by considering the last time you ate—if it's been several hours, it might be genuine hunger. Pay attention to physical signs such as stomach growling or energy depletion. Conversely, if you feel compelled to eat shortly after a meal and your desire is tied to a particular type of food, this may indicate a craving.

Reflect on how emotions or situations are contributing to your urge to eat. If stress or boredom plays a role, acknowledge these feelings without judgment and explore non-food-related responses. Gradually, you'll learn to navigate these triggers with greater ease.

Mindful eating is not about depriving yourself but honoring your body's signals and making thoughtful choices. By distinguishing between hunger and cravings, you'll likely find joy in satisfying genuine hunger while addressing emotional or situational desires outside of food. As you become more attuned to these nuances, the journey toward a balanced lifestyle becomes clearer, paving the way for a healthier relationship with food.

Being Present During Meals to Enhance Satisfaction

When it comes to eating, being fully present can transform an ordinary meal into a richer and more satisfying experience. Mindful consumption invites us to pay attention, genuinely focusing on the food in front of us. This approach enhances the enjoyment we derive from eating and our overall sense of satisfaction. Imagine sitting down to a meal with all your senses engaged—relishing the food's sight, smell, taste, and texture. It's about experiencing meals in a more profound way, where each bite becomes a moment worth savoring.

A key aspect of mindful eating is reducing distractions. In today's fast-paced world, it's easy to find ourselves eating with one hand while scrolling through our phones or watching television. Eliminating such distractions during meals shifts our attention back to eating itself. It encourages us to connect more deeply with the people around us if we're dining with others or with the food and our thoughts if we're alone. This undistracted environment fosters attentive dining, allowing us to appreciate the flavors and textures fully and perhaps even engage in meaningful conversations.

Another technique to deepen our appreciation for meals is slow chewing. By taking the time to chew slowly, we develop a fuller appreciation for the complex flavors many foods offer. Slow chewing is like hitting the pause button, making us more aware of our body's hunger signals. This pace helps control portions naturally because it gives our brains enough time to register when we've eaten enough, aligning with the mindful principle of not overeating.

Moreover, after a meal, reflective practices can play a vital role in how we perceive our eating habits. Considering how the meal made us feel physically and emotionally can help foster a deeper connection with our dietary choices. Did the meal satisfy us, or was there an unmet emotional need? Reflecting on these questions encourages us to make conscious, thoughtful decisions about our diet moving forward.

Incorporating these mindful eating techniques doesn't require drastic changes to our daily routines. It's about making minor adjustments that lead to greater awareness and enjoyment. For example, setting aside a specific portion of time for meals, just as you would for any meaningful activity, creates a dedicated space for mindful eating. You might begin this practice with just one meal daily, focusing on it without interruptions. Over time, this dedication to being present can become part of every meal, leading to a more balanced lifestyle.

The beauty of mindful consumption lies in its simplicity. It's about stripping away the unnecessary layers of distraction and chaos that often surround our mealtimes. Doing so allows us to open ourselves up to a more prosperous, more rewarding relationship with food, driven by genuine appreciation rather than autopilot habits. The interplay between food and mindfulness can be transformative, helping us to appreciate the foods we eat and the occasions and surroundings in which we enjoy them.

Integrating these mindful practices requires patience and persistence. Initially, the challenge may lie in changing ingrained habits of distracted eating. However, the benefits are well worth the effort, offering a pathway to a healthier relationship with food and, ultimately, oneself. A mindful approach to eating allows us to be more attuned to our bodies' natural processes and needs, promoting a sense of balance and well-being beyond the table.

Importantly, mindful eating is a personal journey. There are no strict rules, only guidelines that each person can adapt to fit their lifestyle and needs. What works for one individual might differ for another. The essence of mindful consumption is personalization and attentiveness to one's body and experiences. Whether you're experimenting with reflecting post-meal or practicing gratitude before eating, what matters most is the intention to be present and engaged.

Ultimately, embracing mindful eating isn't about imposing restrictions but liberation from mindless patterns. It's about enjoying food, celebrating its sensory delights, and appreciating the social aspects when dining with others. Each meal becomes a mini-celebration, an opportunity to connect with yourself, your surroundings, and those around you. In this celebration, we find moderation—not through denial or discipline, but genuine, unhurried enjoyment and an understanding of satiety that respects our body's cues.

Moderation as a Tool for Better Digestion

Eating in moderation is more of an art than a science, and it's a skill that significantly influences our digestion and overall health. One key aspect of moderation is understanding portion sizes. Many of us have been conditioned to finish everything on our plates, regardless of how full we might feel. This often leads to discomfort and digestive issues as the stomach struggles to process more food than it can handle effectively. By learning what constitutes a healthy portion size, we allow ourselves to eat enough for satisfaction without overwhelming our digestion. For instance, when you opt for a smaller plate or consciously choose a reasonable serving size, your digestive system can work at its best, leaving you feeling comfortable instead of bloated.

Listening to our body's signals about fullness is another crucial component. Our bodies are equipped with built-in indicators of hunger and satiety, yet in the hustle of modern life, we often override these signals. The concept of Hara Hachi Bu, originating from Okinawa, Japan, advocates eating until you're about 80% full. This practice encourages us to pause and assess our hunger level throughout a meal, promoting mindful decisions about when to stop eating. Listening to these signals prevents overeating and aligns with natural body rhythms, contributing to better digestion and energy balance. It's a gentle reminder that our bodies know best if we take a moment to listen.

Another aspect of moderation is diversity in food choices. It's easy to fall into the trap of routine, consuming the same foods repeatedly. Yet, our bodies thrive on variety, which brings a range of nutrients necessary for optimal health. By diversifying what we eat while practicing moderation, we can ensure that our meals are nutritionally comprehensive and engaging. Think of it as painting with a complete palette rather than just one color; this prevents nutritional deficiencies and keeps mealtimes exciting and satisfying. Including different textures, flavors, and colors can transform eating from a chore into an enjoyable experience while adhering to mindful portions.

The relationship between the amount of food consumed and digestive health cannot be overstated. Our digestive systems, much like any other part of our body, have limits. Over-taxing them with excessive amounts of food can lead to long-term issues such as indigestion, heartburn, or more severe gastrointestinal problems. Conversely, aligning our eating habits with moderate consumption supports our digestive system's ability to function efficiently. This means less strain during breakdown and absorption processes, improving nutrient utilization and overall well-being. With conscious effort and observation, individuals can notice changes in how they feel after altering their portion sizes and food choices.

Ultimately, exploring these principles of moderation equips us with the knowledge to make better long-term dietary decisions. When we understand how what—and how much—we eat affects digestion, we empower ourselves to adopt healthier lifestyles that contribute to longevity and vitality. Choosing moderation doesn't mean deprivation; it's about making informed and balanced choices that cater to our body's needs.

We create a holistic approach to eating by considering all these elements—portion size awareness, intuitive listening to hunger signals, diverse diet choices, and understanding the food-digestion connection. This approach nurtures not just physical health but also mental and emotional well-being by removing guilt and discomfort associated with eating. As adults, particularly those 25 and older, who are more attuned to lifestyle impacts on health, embracing these strategies can significantly improve quality of life. It's a subtle shift in perspective that reaps substantial benefits, transforming meals into acts of self-care and nourishment rather than mere sustenance.

Concluding Thoughts

As we journey through the principles of mindful eating and their intersection with Hara Hachi Bu, we've uncovered the significance of distinguishing between hunger and cravings. This awareness fosters a healthier relationship with food and paves the way for achieving balance in everyday life. By paying attention to our body's signals, we can make more informed choices about what and when to eat, leading to satisfaction that isn't just physical but emotional as well. Practicing these mindful techniques enhances our dining experiences, turning meals into moments of genuine presence and enjoyment.

Furthermore, embracing moderation as a core tool helps us achieve better digestive health and overall well-being. The art of portion control, intuitive listening, and diverse food choices allow us to savor each meal fully without overindulging. It's a gentle reminder that meals should be acts of nourishment and self-care rather than hurried routines. As these practices become natural parts of our daily lives, we nourish our bodies effectively and cultivate a lasting sense of harmony and joy in our eating habits.

31

"You only live once."

Japanese proverb

Chapter 3

Health Benefits of Eating Less

Eating less can be more beneficial to your health than you might think. In a world where portion sizes continue to grow, the ancient practice of Hara Hachi Bu—eating until you're 80% full—offers an alternative path to eating that promotes balance and well-being. This approach, steeped in tradition and supported by current scientific research, challenges our often-mindless consumption patterns. Imagine feeling energized, without the discomfort accompanying overeating, as you embrace a lifestyle that may extend your years. The simplicity of eating until you're not quite full can lead to profound effects on how our bodies function daily. While eating less may sound restricting initially, it's about tuning into natural hunger cues and rediscovering the pleasure of mindful eating.

This chapter delves into the fascinating impact that moderating food intake has on our metabolic processes. We'll explore how adopting practices like Hara Hachi Bu can redefine energy use in your body, making you feel more alert and alive. You'll discover the science behind basal metabolic rate improvements and learn how stabilizing insulin levels can transform sugar metabolism for better weight management. By reducing food intake, your body can shift its focus towards utilizing fat reserves and maintaining lean muscle mass while improving overall energy efficiency. Additionally, we'll examine evidence from communities known for their exceptional longevity, such as those who practice this in Okinawa, demonstrating significant reductions in obesity-related diseases. Through real-world examples and insights, you'll see how small, consistent changes in eating habits are vital to unlocking these health benefits. From enhanced metabolism to sustained energy levels, this chapter offers a roadmap to healthier living, driven by the simple principle of eating a little less.

Impact on Metabolic Processes

In today's fast-paced world, many of us overlook the impact of our eating habits on our bodies. However, adopting practices like Hara Hachi Bu, where one eats until they're about 80% full, can be a game-changer for our metabolic functions and overall energy balance. Let's explore how eating less can influence your body in some incredible ways.

Firstly, when we talk about metabolic processes, the Basal Metabolic Rate (BMR) plays a crucial role in determining how efficiently our body uses energy. Interestingly, reducing caloric intake can improve BMR. This improvement happens because the body adapts to use available resources more efficiently, focusing on maintaining vital functions while storing less energy as fat. For example, if you consume fewer calories than your body needs for basic functioning, it begins optimizing its operations—like a well-tuned machine—to ensure every calorie is used.

Beyond improving efficiency, stabilizing insulin levels becomes achievable with reduced food intake. Consuming large meals frequently often leads to spikes in blood sugar levels, prompting the pancreas to release insulin rapidly. By eating less and more moderately, those spikes become less dramatic, allowing insulin to work more effectively at breaking down sugars. This improved sugar metabolism means glucose is used more readily for energy rather than being converted to fat, contributing to better weight management and metabolic health.

Moreover, by engaging in a lifestyle where caloric consumption is decreased, the body focuses on utilizing stored fat as a primary energy source. This physiological shift occurs because when fewer carbohydrates are burned for immediate energy, the body taps into fat reserves for fuel. It's akin to switching from a quick-burn to a slow-burn energy source, which helps in shedding excess fat and preserves lean muscle mass. People who practice mindful eating often feel more energized and less sluggish as their body's energy demands are steadily met over time.

Improved basal metabolic rates contribute significantly to easier weight management. You might wonder why this is noteworthy. With a higher BMR, the body burns more calories at rest compared to someone with a lower BMR. This means maintaining or achieving a healthy weight becomes more attainable without drastic diet changes or intense exercise regimens. It's like having a head start in a marathon; you cover more ground effortlessly.

Consider this: in regions known for longevity, such as Okinawa, Japan, where Hara Hachi Bu is practiced, there's a noticeably lower prevalence of obesity-related diseases. People adopt a naturally balanced energy allocation by consuming fewer calories, which keeps their BMR active and influential throughout their lives. Their way of life is a testament to how minor adjustments in our eating habits can lead to profound health benefits.

Through these insights, it's clear that eating less doesn't just help you maintain a desirable weight—it fundamentally alters how your body processes energy and nutrients. By improving BMR and encouraging more efficient insulin function, caloric reduction supports a harmonious balance between energy intake and expenditure. Additionally, making a conscious decision to eat less leads your body to more judiciously utilize stored fat, promoting a steady supply of energy and assisting in weight regulation.

Reducing Risks of Chronic Diseases

Eating less, mainly through mindful eating practices like Hara Hachi Bu, offers a variety of health benefits, one of which is significantly reducing the risk associated with chronic diseases. Focusing on consuming fewer calories sets off a domino effect that positively impacts various aspects of our health. Let's delve into these effects to understand how a mindful approach to eating can mitigate potential health threats.

First and foremost, cardiovascular health sees substantial improvement when caloric intake is reduced. Lower calorie consumption has been directly linked to decreased blood pressure and cholesterol levels. Blood pressure is a vital marker of heart health, and high levels often indicate stress on the cardiovascular system. By consuming fewer calories, individuals tend to feel a relaxation in their blood vessels, leading to lower blood pressure. Similarly, cholesterol levels tend to benefit from reduced intake. Bad cholesterol or LDL can be managed more effectively by moderating food intake, thereby decreasing the likelihood of plaque buildup in arteries—a precursor to heart disease. Lifestyle adjustments such as incorporating regular exercise, focusing on whole foods, and reducing portion sizes can further enhance these benefits.

Moving onto diabetes prevention, cutting down on calories is instrumental in managing insulin resistance. Insulin resistance occurs when cells in muscles, fat, and the liver resist or ignore the signal insulin sends—which can lead to Type 2 diabetes. Studies have shown that a mindful eating approach can help maintain stable blood sugar levels, thus lowering insulin resistance. By eating less, the body's need to produce massive amounts of insulin decreases, improving its sensitivity to this hormone over time. This means less strain on the pancreas and better overall metabolic health.

Caloric restriction also shows promising results in reducing cancer risks. Chronic inflammation contributes to the development of certain cancers; it is aggravated by obesity and high caloric intake. Eating less can prevent excessive inflammation, thereby reducing cancer risks. Research indicates that individuals who follow caloric restriction can enjoy lowered markers of inflammation. This preventive measure works best with a diet rich in antioxidants—such as fruits, vegetables, nuts, and seeds—that help fight inflammation head-on.

In addition to these benefits, joint and bone health significantly improve with moderated caloric intake. Overweight individuals often experience additional pressure on their joints, leading to conditions like osteoarthritis. Excess body weight increases mechanical load and accelerates joint wear and tear. By consuming fewer calories and maintaining a balanced weight, the pressure exerted on joints diminishes, reducing pain and the risk of developing arthritis. This improvement extends to enhanced bone health, as moderate body weight supports the bones' structural integrity without overwhelming them. Strength-training exercises and mindful eating can provide even greater joint and bone health sustenance.

Mindful eating, as emphasized in the Hara Hachi Bu practice, requires us to eat slowly and stop when satisfied but not completely. This approach encourages paying attention to hunger cues, savoring each bite, and aligning eating habits with our body's genuine needs—all of which contribute to the positive outcomes discussed above. It's not merely about eating less; it's about eating consciously and making informed dietary choices.

Improving Mental Clarity and Energy Levels

Eating less can significantly enhance cognitive performance, a benefit rooted in ancient wisdom and modern science. The notion that reducing food intake improves memory and attention span is supported by numerous studies, revealing fascinating insights into how our brains respond to caloric intake. For instance, research suggests that a lighter diet can increase the production of brain-derived neurotrophic factor (BDNF), a protein crucial for long-term memory and learning. This means that when we eat just enough to satisfy our hunger and not indulge beyond that, we nourish our bodies and support mental sharpness.

Consider a real-world application—how often have you experienced that sleepy, sluggish feeling after a big meal? Your body directs energy towards digestion, leaving less for brain activity. By eating until 80% full, known as Hara Hachi Bu, we can allocate more energy to maintain alertness and focus. This restraint doesn't mean deprivation; instead, it allows the body to operate more efficiently, ensuring that energy is available for critical thinking and problem-solving. In workplaces or study environments, where concentration is paramount, this slight adjustment in eating habits could lead to noticeable improvements in productivity and attentiveness.

Overeating directly correlates with fatigue, a fact often overlooked in discussions about diet and health. When we consume more food than necessary, the body must work overtime to digest and process it, leaving us drained and lethargic. In contrast, when we moderate our consumption, we sustain higher energy levels throughout the day. Imagine approaching daily tasks with a reservoir of vitality rather than battling the mid-afternoon slump— a common predicament caused by indulgence in heavy lunches. Keeping meals lighter and portion-controlled helps avoid this energy dip, empowering individuals to remain active and engaged from morning to evening.

The relationship between caloric moderation and mood stability is intricate yet pivotal. Serotonin, often dubbed the "feel-good" neurotransmitter, regulates our mood and well-being. It's synthesized in the brain and heavily influenced by what and how much we eat. Overconsumption can disrupt serotonin balance, possibly leading to mood swings and irritability. However, when we eat in moderation, serotonin levels stabilize, promoting emotional equilibrium. Those who adopt this mindful approach often find themselves experiencing fewer mood fluctuations and maintaining a more consistent sense of happiness and calm throughout the day.

Streamlined digestion from eating less offers the remarkable benefit of making one feel lighter and more active—a sensation anyone can appreciate. When an excess of food doesn't bog down the digestive system, it can operate more smoothly, resulting in increased energy availability for other physical activities. Whether going for a brisk walk, working out, or simply completing everyday chores, this enhanced vitality promotes overall wellness and reduces the feeling of being weighed down. Furthermore, efficient digestion positively impacts nutrient absorption, ensuring that our bodies benefit from the nutrients consumed, which further supports our active lifestyles.

A clear guideline for preventing mental fog is structuring meals around moderation. Begin by listening to your body's innate signals of hunger and fullness, something many of us have become disconnected from in pursuit of oversized portions. Practicing mindful eating—savoring each bite, recognizing satisfaction over satiety—can gradually recalibrate these signals. Setting smaller portions and pausing during meals can clarify if additional food is necessary. Over time, this habit can prevent the mental fog associated with excessive food intake, leading to sharper cognitive abilities.

In addition to practical strategies, historical contexts, and cultural practices reinforce the benefits of eating less. Many societies, particularly in Asia, have long embraced principles akin to Hara Hachi Bu. This traditional wisdom underscores the understanding that dietary habits are interconnected with longevity and high quality of life. Studying populations adhering to these ideologies reveals lower incidences of age-related cognitive decline, serving as a powerful testament to the profound impact of our eating choices on brain health.

Focusing on caloric moderation may help individuals better handle stress and challenges. With stable serotonin levels and improved mood regulation, responses to external pressures become more measured and effective. This aspect of emotional resilience is invaluable in today's fast-paced world, where stress management is vital to personal and professional success. It offers a sustainable way to combat stress-induced eating behaviors, creating a positive feedback loop that enhances psychological well-being.

Finally, integrating these dietary changes doesn't necessitate drastic lifestyle overhauls. Simple steps like choosing nutrient-dense foods, prioritizing vegetables and lean proteins, and avoiding sugary snacks can gently guide one toward eating less without feeling deprived. Embracing the principle of eating until moderately full encourages a focus on nutrient quality over quantity, maximizing health benefits and fostering a balanced approach to nourishment.

Final Thoughts

By exploring the benefits of Hara Hachi Bu, we have ventured into a world where eating less can transform not just our bodies but also our minds and spirits. As we've seen, this practice prioritizes metabolic efficiency and encourages a harmonious dance between energy intake and expenditure. Embracing the wisdom embedded in eating until 80% full, you set off a chain reaction that enhances basal metabolic rates and insulin functionality. This helps manage weight, paves the way for improved cardiovascular health, and reduces risks associated with chronic conditions like diabetes and cancer. It's about creating a nutritional balance that aligns with your body's needs—leading to a healthier and more vibrant life.

Beyond physical health, the principles of Hara Hachi Bu ripple through mental clarity and emotional well-being. Consuming moderate portions stabilizes mood, sharpens focus, and empowers you with sustained energy levels throughout the day. This mindful approach to eating allows you to remain alert and engaged, transforming daily routines and interactions. By tuning into hunger cues and savoring each bite, you're reconnecting with your natural rhythm, fostering a sense of balance across body and mind. As you incorporate these practices into your lifestyle, you're honoring a tradition backed by science and nurturing a path toward longevity and fulfillment.

"It is the effort that makes the
impossible possible."

Japanese proverb

Chapter 4

Integrating Hara Hachi Bu in Daily Life

Integrating Hara Hachi Bu into daily life involves adopting mindful eating strategies that focus on eating until you're about 80% full. This ancient Japanese practice encourages individuals to develop a keen awareness of their body's hunger and fullness cues, promoting health and longevity naturally. While it may seem simple at first glance, the philosophy requires a shift in how we perceive food and eating habits. By allowing oneself to stop eating just before reaching complete satiety, one can avoid the discomfort of overindulgence and prevent future health issues associated with overeating. Such an approach respects the body's natural signals and aligns with modern understandings of balanced nutrition.

This chapter will delve into practical strategies for successfully incorporating Hara Hachi Bu into your routine. Readers will discover how setting personal boundaries can help align their eating habits with health objectives, fostering self-discipline and mindfulness. The text will explore various methods for defining these boundaries, such as recognizing triggers of mindless eating and using smaller dishes to manage portion sizes. Additionally, the concept of making incremental changes—rather than drastic overnight shifts—will be covered, offering manageable steps toward embodying this philosophy. Furthermore, the chapter highlights the benefits of journaling for enhancing self-awareness and accountability in pursuing mindful eating. Finally, readers will learn the importance of celebrating achievements and creating positive associations with mindful eating, motivating them to continue integrating Hara Hachi Bu into everyday life. By the end of this chapter, you will have actionable insights and techniques to cultivate more mindful and health-conscious eating habits aligned with Hara Hachi Bu principles.

Setting Practical Goals for Mindful Eating

Defining personal boundaries is a critical step in integrating the Hara Hachi Bu philosophy into daily life, as it aids in aligning eating habits with one's health objectives. By setting clear limits on portion sizes and meal times, individuals can foster self-discipline and develop a more mindful approach to eating. For example, they decide to stop eating when 80% full aligns perfectly with this philosophy, allowing the body to signal proper fullness without overindulgence. These boundaries not only help in managing portion sizes but also encourage an introspective look into what your body's needs are versus habitual or emotional eating triggers.

Guidelines for defining personal boundaries include identifying situations where you often overeat or consume food mindlessly. Once identified, create specific rules for those moments, such as portioning food before eating or using smaller dishes to limit intake naturally. Practicing these boundaries consistently encourages adherence to mindful eating practices, reinforcing the connection between what you eat and how it impacts your health.

Creating incremental changes is another essential strategy in applying Hara Hachi Bu to daily life. Rather than completely overhauling one's dietary habits overnight, focusing on minor, gradual adjustments is more sustainable and manageable. For instance, gradually reducing portions or slowly incorporating more plant-based foods into meals can be practical starting points. This method respects the natural resistance many have to drastic change and instead celebrates small victories that collectively lead to significant progress.

To effectively create incremental changes, start with simple actions such as swapping a sugary snack for a piece of fruit or cutting down on unnecessary second helpings during meals. Document these changes and recognize their positive effects on your health and well-being. Over time, these minor alterations accumulate, leading to significant improvements in eating habits without feeling deprivation or restriction. Thus, they build resilience and foster a mindset geared towards long-term success.

Journaling progress is a powerful tool for enhancing self-awareness, accountability, and motivation. By keeping track of what and how much you eat, along with your thoughts and feelings during meals, you create a dynamic record that offers insights into eating patterns and triggers. This reflective practice can help identify areas for improvement and highlight successful strategies already in place.

A guideline for effective journaling might involve keeping a daily log of your meals, including the time, place, and portion sizes consumed. Remember to note emotional cues, stress levels, or social contexts, as these factors often influence eating behaviors. Reviewing these entries can clarify personal progress and motivate you to stay committed to the goals set. Seeing tangible evidence of mindful eating successes can boost confidence and reinforce dedication to maintaining these new habits.

Celebrating achievements is vital to sustaining motivation and commitment to mindful eating regardless of size. Acknowledging and rewarding yourself for reaching milestones—such as consistently stopping when you feel satisfied rather than full—can significantly bolster self-confidence. This positive reinforcement makes it easier to persevere through challenging times when the lure of old habits might resurface.

While it's important not to overindulge in celebratory acts that might counteract your healthy intentions, finding non-food-related ways to celebrate can be particularly effective. Treat yourself to a relaxing activity, buy a new book, or enjoy leisure time pursuing a hobby. By associating joy and reward with progress in mindful eating, you're building a more substantial commitment to continue integrating the principles of Hara Hachi Bu into everyday life.

Adapting Meal Portions at Home and Dining Out

Incorporating the Hara Hachi Bu philosophy into daily life involves adopting practical strategies for mindful eating, and managing portion sizes is a crucial aspect of this process. One effective technique to regulate portions is using smaller plates. Research suggests that we tend to fill our plates to the brim, regardless of their size. By choosing smaller dishes, we naturally reduce the food we serve ourselves. This method works by leveraging the Delboeuf illusion, a psychological phenomenon where the same quantity of food appears more substantial on a smaller plate than on a larger one. As a result, individuals are more likely to feel satisfied with less food, promoting fullness without the temptation to overeat. Implementing this straightforward change in tableware can guide us toward consuming fewer calories while enjoying our meals.

Transitioning from individual dining experiences to shared ones, serving meals family-style also offers benefits in controlling portion sizes. In this setup, food is placed in dishes on the table, and people help themselves, encouraging them to take only what they need. This practice fosters a sense of moderation as everyone becomes more conscious of selecting appropriate portions. Moreover, it enhances the dining experience by facilitating interaction among diners, transforming meals into enjoyable social occasions rather than mere acts of consumption. By being mindful of how much food makes it onto their plates, individuals can better align their eating habits with the principles of Hara Hachi Bu, prioritizing satisfaction over sheer volume.

Navigating menus effectively is another critical skill for managing portions, especially dining out. Many restaurants serve huge meals, which can lead to unintended caloric overspending. To combat this, it's helpful to employ specific techniques when ordering. Start by scanning the menu for dishes that feature lean proteins and vegetables, as these often provide balance without excessive calories. Additionally, consider sharing entrees or opting for appetizers as mains to decrease portion sizes. It's also helpful to ask questions about preparation methods, such as whether foods are grilled instead of fried, which can significantly impact the overall caloric content of a dish. By honing these menu navigation skills, diners can make informed choices that adhere to the Hara Hachi Bu philosophy even outside the home environment.

Asking for meal modifications plays a vital role in controlling portion sizes. This approach requires a proactive mindset where diners are encouraged to customize their orders to suit their dietary preferences and portion needs better. Simple requests like asking for dressings or sauces on the side, substituting fries for a salad, or requesting half portions demonstrate an awareness of personal health goals. Such adjustments aid in managing intake and set an example for others, encouraging them to take similar steps towards mindful eating. By advocating for their needs in a restaurant setting, individuals become more attuned to their hunger cues and reinforce the importance of eating until 80% full—a core tenet of Hara Hachi Bu.

Guided by these strategies, readers can embrace the art of portion control as a seamless part of their routine. Utilizing smaller plates, for instance, can be easily implemented at home. It presents minimal disruption to daily life while offering significant benefits in reducing overall food consumption. Similarly, experimenting with family-style dining could become an engaging way to involve family and friends in mindful eating. Encouraging open discussion about portion preferences during meals can lead to more supportive environments where everyone feels comfortable taking what they need and leaving behind excess.

Engaging with menus and voicing modification requests in restaurant settings equips individuals with the confidence to make healthier choices. These practices reinforce autonomy over one's diet, leading to greater dining satisfaction. Rather than viewing restaurant portions as obligatory servings, diners can feel empowered to shape their meals to fit their health objectives.

Overcoming Societal Pressures to Overeat

Navigating social situations that encourage overeating can be quite a challenge, as it often involves a mix of external pressures and internal motivations. It is easy to find oneself swayed by social cues that pull us toward another helping or an extra slice of dessert. Recognizing these cues is the first step towards mindful eating. At gatherings, there may be subtle expectations to partake in multiple servings or try every dish out of politeness or tradition. By becoming more conscious of these societal norms, individuals can identify moments when they're about to eat not out of hunger but to meet unspoken social obligations.

Understanding these dynamics enables individuals to practice mindfulness during social engagements. Mindfulness begins with awareness, and awareness starts with recognizing specific triggers that lead to overeating. These can include the sight of abundant food, the smell wafting from a buffet table, or even the joyful laughter of people enjoying their meals. Once you notice these triggers, it becomes easier to step back and decide whether your next bite is aligned with your health goals rather than just conforming to social pressures.

Another effective strategy is setting intentions before attending any gathering. This practice involves taking time before the event to reflect on how you wish to engage with the food offered. Setting intentions could mean deciding that you'll enjoy one serving of a particular dish or savor a dessert mindfully without indulging in seconds. Establishing these intentions beforehand creates a mental framework that supports mindful decisions, even amidst the chaos and allure of social dining.

There are several guidelines to support this intention-setting process. Firstly, visualize the event and the types of foods that will likely be available. Consider what you genuinely want to taste and create a mental plan to enjoy these choices in moderation. Secondly, remind yourself of past scenarios where you've felt guilt or discomfort after overeating. Use these memories as gentle nudges to stick with your intentions. Lastly, share your plans with a supportive friend who might also be attending. Having someone else aware of your intentions can provide extra accountability and encouragement.

Redirecting focus from food to connection through meaningful conversations is equally crucial in navigating these situations. Social events offer invaluable opportunities to deepen relationships and form new ones, and engaging in conversations can be a pleasant distraction from the abundance of food. Initiate discussions on topics that interest you and those around you, which naturally diverts attention away from how much everyone eats.

Engaging deeply with others enhances the quality of your social experience and shifts the focus from the quantity of food consumed to the richness of the interactions shared. It's a beautiful way to cultivate genuine connections while subtly reinforcing control over your eating habits. Moreover, participating actively in conversations provides the additional benefit of slowing down your eating pace, allowing you to better tune into your body's satiety signals.

A tactful yet assertive approach to maintaining personal dietary boundaries involves practicing polite declines. This means feeling confident enough to say no to additional servings or politely declining food offers without feeling guilty or offending anyone. While declining may feel uncomfortable initially, understanding that it's an expression of personal autonomy helps reinforce that such boundaries are essential for one's well-being.

Guidelines for practicing polite declines can make this process smoother. Start by expressing appreciation for the offer—something as simple as "Thank you, that looks delicious!" shows respect and gratitude. Follow this with a straightforward but courteous explanation, such as "I'm trying to watch my portions tonight," or "No, thank you, I'm full." Being firm yet respectful indicates your resolution without inviting further persuasion. Over time, this assertion becomes second nature, affirming your commitment to mindful eating regardless of the situation.

Bringing It All Together

This chapter explores practical strategies for incorporating the Hara Hachi Bu philosophy into our daily lives to cultivate mindful eating habits. Individuals can align their eating habits with health objectives by setting personal boundaries and making incremental changes without feeling overwhelmed. Whether choosing smaller plates at home or navigating restaurant menus mindfully, these approaches emphasize portion control, allowing us to truly enjoy our meals without overeating. Journaling emerges as a vital tool for self-awareness and motivation, offering insights into our eating patterns and highlighting successes. Celebrating milestones, no matter how small, is essential in maintaining enthusiasm and commitment to these new habits.

Mindful eating is not just about food; it involves understanding societal pressures and making intentional choices in social settings. Recognizing triggers and setting intentions before gatherings supports mindful decision-making while redirecting focus from food to meaningful interactions, which enhances our social experiences and helps maintain dietary goals. Practicing polite declines empowers us to stay true to our boundaries without guilt. Through these strategies, we embrace the art of mindful eating, striving for satisfaction and well-being, ultimately fostering a healthier relationship with food that aligns with the Hara Hachi Bu philosophy.

57

> "Only staying active will make you
> want to live a hundred years."
>
> Japanese proverb

Chapter 5

A Culinary Journey Through Okinawa

Embarking on a culinary journey through Okinawa offers the opportunity to delve into a world of vibrant flavors and time-honored traditions. Renowned for its unique approach to food, Okinawan cuisine emphasizes balance, nutrition, and mindful eating. Rooted deeply in the principle of Hara Hachi Bu, which encourages consuming food until one is only 80% full, these practices illuminate the path towards longevity and wellness that Okinawans have cherished for generations. This chapter promises an expedition into the heart of Okinawan kitchens, where every ingredient tells a story, and every dish celebrates nature's bounty.

Throughout this exploration, we'll dive into nutrient-rich staples, each chosen for their taste and health benefits. Expect to discover how sweet potatoes, with their vivid colors, serve more than just visual appeal. At the same time, bitter melon challenges the palate with its distinct taste yet rewards it with nutritional power. We'll also embrace the beauty of traditional recipes like Okinawan Soba and Miso Soup, which masterfully balance ingredients within the framework of Hara Hachi Bu. Furthermore, the chapter sheds light on Okinawa's practice of seasonal eating—a tradition that harmonizes with nature's rhythms and speaks volumes about sustainable living. As we uncover these culinary secrets, readers are invited to appreciate the simplicity and depth of Okinawan dishes and their philosophies.

Nutrient-Rich Okinawan Ingredients

When you think of Okinawan cuisine, one of the first images that might come to mind is the brightly colored sweet potato. This staple has deep roots in the culture and offers more than just vibrant hues. Sweet potatoes in Okinawa are known for stabilizing blood sugar levels. This is mainly due to their low glycemic index, meaning they release glucose slowly into the bloodstream. Not only do these tubers provide sustained energy, but they also pack a punch with a rich array of vitamins, including vitamins A and C. These nutrients play a role in maintaining healthy skin and boosting the immune system, making sweet potatoes an integral part of mindful eating practices.

Now, let's move from underground to above ground, where leafy greens like Goya, known as bitter melon, take center stage. Goya's distinctive flavor might be an acquired taste, but its nutritional benefits are undeniable. It's rich in vitamins and minerals, particularly vitamin C and folate, which enhance dietary diversity. What's remarkable about Goya is that despite being nutrient-dense, it is low in calories. This makes it a perfect choice for those seeking a healthy diet without consuming excess calories. Incorporating leafy greens such as Goya into meals adds variety and supports the body's overall well-being.

Fish is another cornerstone of the Okinawan diet, serving as a primary source of protein. With coastal access, Okinawans have long relied on seafood, rich in omega-3 fatty acids, essential for promoting heart health. Regular fish consumption aligns seamlessly with the principles of moderation championed by the cultural practice of Hara Hachi Bu—eating until you're 80% full. This moderate approach ensures that individuals benefit from the rich nutrients found in seafood, such as DHA and EPA, which contribute to cardiovascular health and cognitive function without overindulging.

Soy products are unique in Okinawan meals, offering plant-based protein with minimal saturated fat content. Foods like tofu and miso are versatile and easy to digest, making them excellent choices for balanced eating. Soy isoflavones found abundantly in these products have been associated with various health benefits, including improved digestion and reduced risk of certain chronic diseases. By replacing some animal proteins with soy products, individuals can reduce their intake of unhealthy fats while still enjoying satisfying, protein-rich meals.

Traditional Recipes That Emphasize Balance

Okinawan cuisine is renowned for its balance and nutritional wholeness, making it a fascinating culinary art to explore—primarily through the practice of Hara Hachi Bu. At the heart of this cultural approach to eating is Okinawan Soba. This dish isn't just about taste; it's a masterful blend of carbohydrates, proteins, and vegetables in one bowl. Made using buckwheat noodles, tofu, and seasonal vegetables, Okinawan Soba offers a fulfilling meal that respects the 80% rule—eating until you're only 80% full. It's a great example of a balanced diet, savoring the nutrient-rich traditions of Okinawa while being mindful of moderation.

The versatility of Okinawan Soba allows for ample experimentation with various ingredients. For instance, substituting pork or adding seafood can bring different textures and flavors, keeping the dish exciting without straying from its essence. The journey doesn't end at creativity; it extends to the health benefits. Buckwheat noodles are a source of complex carbohydrates, providing sustained energy throughout the day. Tofu complements this by offering lean protein for muscle repair and growth, while vegetables add vitamins and minerals vital for overall health.

Transitioning from soba to another staple, Miso Soup is a beloved part of the Okinawan diet, symbolizing warmth and nourishment. More than just a comfort food, Miso Soup is rich in probiotics, which play an essential role in promoting gut health. These beneficial bacteria help maintain a healthy digestive system, which is crucial for nutrient absorption and immune function. What makes Miso Soup truly special is its encouragement of using leftovers creatively. Almost any vegetable or protein can be added to this base, providing endless variations while minimizing waste.

Incorporating leftovers into Miso Soup reflects the Okinawan philosophy of respecting food resources and appreciating what's available. The soup symbolizes a harmonious melding of flavors and cultures as you combine the ingredients. By customizing each bowl according to personal preference or seasonal availability, Miso Soup becomes more than a meal—an expression of individuality and innovation in the kitchen.

Then there's Goya Chanpuru, an iconic dish for its unique combination of protein and vegetables in a stir-fry format. Bitter melon, or Goya, provides a distinct flavor profile that challenges traditional Western palates. Yet, its bitterness is worth embracing. Rich in antioxidants and nutrients, Goya improves digestion and reduces blood sugar levels. Pairing it with tofu and pork creates a delightful contrast of crisp, soft, and tender textures.

A quick stir-fry of Goya Chanpuru ensures that the natural flavors and nutrients remain intact. This efficient cooking method aligns well with busy lifestyles while meeting dietary needs. Eating Goya Chanpuru can be a reminder of the importance of embracing diverse tastes and enjoying the nutritious bounty that nature provides, even those that may initially seem unfamiliar or unconventional.

Finally, Chirashizushi is a beautiful embodiment of visually and nutritionally balanced food. Also known as scattered sushi, this dish features vinegared rice adorned with a rainbow of ingredients like sliced fish, vegetables, and eggs. Its vibrant appearance isn't just for show—it reflects a meal that balances elements meticulously. The rice, a staple carbohydrate, grounds the dish, while the variety of toppings provides essential proteins and micronutrients.

Chirashizushi invites personalization, allowing diners to select their favorite ingredients and explore new combinations. Unlike a canvas, each preparation feels like a work of art tailored to the individual, while meditative meal preparation nurtures mindfulness. Crafting Chirashizushi fosters a deeper appreciation of food, the processes involved in producing it, and its role in sustaining us physically and emotionally.

Seasonal Eating in Okinawa

In the vibrant landscape of Okinawa, seasonal eating is much more than just a dietary choice; it's a way of life. As the seasons shift, so too do the fruits and vegetables that grace the tables of this island community. Consuming what nature offers at specific times of the year supports personal health and promotes environmental sustainability. By embracing seasonal harvest practices, Okinawans naturally align with a philosophy of moderation and a deep understanding of their food sources.

Okinawa's tradition of seasonal eating involves savoring produce at its peak when flavors are enhanced and nutritional content is optimal. For example, bitter melon, or Goya, appears in early spring. Known for its distinct taste and myriad health benefits, it's a staple in many local dishes during this time. In summer, mangoes burst into abundance, providing a sweet respite from the heat while delivering essential vitamins. These seasonal delicacies invite individuals to appreciate the natural ebb and flow of the environment, encouraging moderation by dictating availability.

The culinary arts take center stage in Okinawan festivals, which occur yearly. These events are not merely opportunities for celebration but are vital in strengthening community bonds. During these gatherings, shared meals made from locally sourced, seasonal ingredients play a critical role. Imagine families and friends coming together during the autumn festival to share soups brimming with freshly harvested pumpkin, sweet potatoes, and other warm, comforting ingredients. Such meals highlight the importance of health-focused culinary traditions, enhancing physical well-being and social connectivity.

Beyond individual health, seasonal eating dramatically impacts the environment. Consuming locally available foods reduces the carbon footprint of transporting out-of-season produce over long distances. In Okinawa, where agriculture is closely tied to the land and sea, this practice maintains ecological balance and supports the local economy. Fishing communities, for instance, rely on sustainable methods that ensure fish populations remain stable, reflecting a deep respect for natural resources.

The concept of recipe mapping is another fascinating aspect of Okinawan culinary culture. It encourages creativity in meal preparation, guiding cooks to devise recipes in harmony with nature's cycles. A simple yet profound illustration of this is the seasonal adaptation of traditional Okinawan soba noodles. The dish might be enriched in winter with hearty root vegetables and mushrooms, providing warmth and nourishment. Conversely, fresh herbs and citrus could be lightened in summer, offering refreshment and vitality. Recipe mapping ensures that meals are balanced, nutritious, and aligned with sustainability principles.

Okinawans practice intuitive mindfulness by prioritizing seasonal eating and respecting the earth's rhythm. They inherently understand that moderation, as reflected in the principle of Hara Hachi Bu—eating until 80% full—extends beyond personal consumption to include how we interact with our surroundings. This perspective fosters a respectful coexistence with nature, underscoring the importance of making conscious choices about our diets for the health of both ourselves and the planet.

Insights and Implications

Exploring traditional Okinawan foods offers a window into a cultural practice emphasizing health, sustainability, and moderation. At the heart of this exploration lies the vibrant array of nutrient-rich ingredients such as sweet potatoes, bitter melon, fish, and soy products. These foods provide more than sustenance; they embody the Okinawan approach to balanced eating through Hara Hachi Bu—an ethos of consuming until one is 80% full. By appreciating these ingredients' unique benefits, from stabilizing blood sugar to enhancing cardiovascular health, we are reminded of the importance of mindful choices in our diets and how they contribute to overall well-being.

Okinawa's culinary traditions also celebrate the seasons' rhythm, showcasing dishes like Okinawan Soba, Miso Soup, Goya Chanpuru, and Chirashizushi. Each recipe is a testament to balance, creativity, and sustainability, drawing on the freshest seasonal produce. As we savor these flavors, we're encouraged to embrace an appreciation for nature's cycles and our connection to the environment. This chapter invites readers to enjoy the richness of Okinawan cuisine and reflect on the broader implications of how we eat—as individuals and as a community deeply rooted in respect for natural resources.

68

"Keep going; don't change your path."

Mitsuo Aida

Chapter 6

Challenges of Mindful Eating in Modern Times

Mindful eating is a journey that poses unique hurdles in the hustle and bustle of today's world. It's not just about what we eat but how we engage with our meals amidst advertisements, social cues, and emotional undercurrents. Our lives are dominated by fast-moving schedules and digital distractions, making it easy to fall into patterns of mindless munching. Imagine grabbing a quick bite while scrolling through your phone or skipping breakfast because you're late for work. These scenarios highlight the constant tug between intent and practicality. With an awareness of these everyday realities, we can begin to navigate the intricate maze of modern eating habits.

Through this chapter, you will be guided on a thoughtful exploration of the obstacles between us and mindful eating. We'll delve into the impact of rapid lifestyles where convenience often trumps nutrition and the unseen influences of advertisements shaping our cravings. The chapter sheds light on the emotional triggers prompting us to reach for food as comfort rather than nourishment and the persistent peer pressures that linger in social settings. Each section offers insights and practical strategies to help you recognize and overcome these barriers. By understanding the forces at play, you'll gain tools to reclaim control, cultivate mindfulness, and enrich your relationship with food—a rewarding pursuit in today's demanding times.

Dealing with Fast-Paced Lifestyles

Navigating our fast-paced world can make mindful eating feel like an elusive goal. The demands of busy schedules often push us to rely on convenience foods that are quick and easy but only sometimes the healthiest choices. With packed calendars, it's tempting to sacrifice mealtimes to save a few minutes, but this can lead to poor eating habits and diminished well-being. Prioritizing meal times as an essential self-care practice is crucial. By seeing these moments as opportunities to nurture both body and mind, individuals can make more thoughtful food choices, escaping the trap of rushed and careless eating.

Time constraints frequently lead to mindless eating habits. Rushed meals often happen when we need more time to eat with distractions. Setting aside undisturbed time for meals helps cultivate an environment where mindfulness thrives. An effective strategy is to set daily reminders to slow down and savor each bite, even during a busy day. This conscious eating practice allows for better digestion and provides the space to connect with your plate's food. Mindfulness breaks during meals—brief pauses to breathe profoundly or clear your mind—can serve as calm anchors, ensuring a more focused eating experience despite limited time.

Workplace environments pose particular challenges, as food culture within office settings often promotes unhealthy eating due to peer pressure and the constant availability of junk foods. It's expected to be surrounded by snacks laden with sugar and empty calories, shared freely among colleagues. Encouraging healthier snack options in the workplace is essential. Creating a communal fruit bowl or bringing homemade, nutritious snacks can set positive examples for others. Moreover, fostering supportive conversations around mindful eating principles can gradually shift collective attitudes towards food at work, making it a shared priority rather than an individual challenge.

Multitasking while eating is another common habit that can undermine mindfulness. Eating in front of screens — whether working on a computer, watching TV, or scrolling through social media — distracts from the sensory experience of eating. To counteract this, embrace the concept of distraction-free dining. Consider a 'digital detox' during meals to eliminate the urge to multitask. Turning off devices and focusing solely on the meal enhances the pleasure derived from each flavor and texture. Additionally, incorporating practices such as mindful breathing before eating can prime the mind to concentrate fully on the dining experience, ensuring that meals are moments of joy and reflection rather than just another task to complete.

Amidst the busyness of life, planning becomes a powerful ally. Taking time to plan and schedule meals can significantly improve the quality of food choices, enabling healthier decisions even on tight timelines. This might involve meal prepping in advance or setting simple weekly menus. Planning allows you to approach meals intentionally, reducing reliance on unhealthy convenience foods. Batch-cooking strategies also offer a practical solution to time pressures. Preparing large meals beforehand ensures that wholesome, homemade options are always ready, minimizing the need for less nutritious alternatives.

Reminders to eat slowly and intentionally, even on the most hectic days, can foster long-term benefits. In our rush from one task to the next, we risk losing touch with essential cues like hunger and fullness. Simple tools such as phone alarms or calendar alerts can prompt you to pause and check in with yourself, reinforcing the importance of mindful consumption. When meals become mindful pauses in the day, they provide a reprieve from the relentless pace of modern living.

Navigating Through Food Marketing Tactics

In today's fast-paced world, mindfulness in eating often takes a backseat, overshadowed by the numerous marketing strategies vying for our attention. One of the most prevalent tactics used by food marketers is persuasive advertising. These advertisements tap into our emotions, leading to impulsive eating behaviors that conflict with mindful eating practices. Advertisements often use catchy jingles, vibrant imagery, and emotional storytelling to connect with the audience, creating a sense of need rather than want. It's crucial to understand the psychological tactics at play here.

Critical evaluation of food commercials is essential for making informed decisions. Picture yourself walking through a grocery store: bright colors pop from every corner, each product claiming superiority over its competition. When faced with these allurements, it's helpful to pause and reflect on the motivations behind the advertising. Ask yourself what emotions are being targeted. Are these ads making you feel nostalgia, happiness, or excitement? Recognizing these psychological triggers allows you to make more conscious choices that align with your dietary goals.

Convenience stores and packaged foods present another significant challenge to mindful eating. These products are often marketed as quick solutions for busy lives but frequently lack nutritional value. How usually do we pick up a microwave meal without glancing at the ingredient list? Encouraging label reading is not just an act of scrutiny but a step towards reclaiming control over your eating habits. Understanding the ingredients ensures you know what you're consuming, helping you discern healthier options amidst convenience.

But convenience doesn't have to mean unhealthy. There are myriad options available that are both quick to prepare and nutritious. For example, pre-chopped vegetables and ready-to-eat salads offer speed without sacrificing health. Teaching readers to read labels and comprehend ingredient lists empowers them to make healthier choices. Moreover, consider alternatives like overnight oats or fruit smoothies—foods that marry convenience with wholesome goodness, keeping your diet balanced even on tight schedules. Offering alternatives to convenience foods builds a bridge between ease and nourishment.

Balancing convenience with nutritional value demands thoughtful decision-making. This balance can enrich our daily routines, ensuring quick meals don't compromise our well-being. Discussing the balance between convenience and nutritional value is vital for any long-term dietary strategy. Imagine the satisfaction of enjoying a home-cooked meal that was both practical to prepare and rich in nutrients—that's the harmony we're seeking to achieve.

On the digital front, social media significantly influences how we view food. Platforms are rife with unrealistic food ideals, and fleeting trends often contradict mindful eating principles. Curated images of perfect meals can instill feelings of inadequacy or push us towards unsustainable diets. It becomes imperative to curate our feeds thoughtfully, following influencers who promote positive, realistic eating habits.

Developing personal food philosophies is another tool in combating social media's sometimes toxic influence. These philosophies should align with individual values and needs, promoting a healthy relationship with food. They enable you to filter out noise and focus on what's genuinely beneficial, fostering a space where mindful eating can thrive. Curating their feeds to focus on positive, mindful eating messages helps navigate the digital landscape with intention and care.

Finally, we confront the health halo effect. This phenomenon occurs when unhealthy foods are marketed as healthy, misleading even the most careful consumers. Products may boast low fats or sugars while hiding high sodium content or artificial additives. To sidestep such traps, learning to recognize genuine health claims versus deceitful marketing is invaluable.

The key lies in understanding labels and seeking transparency. Is the "low-fat" yogurt compensating with extra sugar? Does this "whole grain" cereal contain negligible fiber? By questioning these claims, you become adept at navigating the maze of food packaging and choosing truly nourishing options. Educating consumers about this can dismantle the health halo illusion, steering them toward authentic well-being.

Handling Emotional Eating Triggers

In today's fast-paced world, emotional eating often creeps into our lives without us even realizing it. We might find ourselves reaching for that chocolate bar or bag of chips not because we're hungry but because emotions are bubbling up—stress from work, loneliness, boredom, or even the lingering aftereffects of a tough day. The first step to tackling this challenge is identifying those emotional triggers that prompt us to eat when we're not physically hungry.

Imagine a moment of stress at work. Instead of automatically reaching for a snack, consider keeping a journal handy. Jot down what you're feeling before diving into that treat. Was it frustration? Anxiety? Happiness? By consistently doing this, patterns emerge, giving you a clearer picture of how emotions intertwine with your eating habits. Mindfulness techniques can also be helpful here; they invite you to pause and honestly assess your feelings, offering a chance to breathe deeply and contemplate whether that hunger is physical or emotional.

Once you've recognized these emotional triggers, developing coping strategies becomes essential. Imagine swapping out comfort food with activities that bring joy and relaxation yet don't involve eating. Try meditation—a few minutes of deep breathing can do wonders and calm your mind. Or perhaps engage in a hobby like painting, playing music, or crafting, which can channel emotional energy into creativity rather than consumption. If emotional eating persists, joining support groups or seeking professional guidance can provide additional support layers, offering avenues to share experiences and learn from others on similar journeys.

Another aspect to consider is self-compassion. It's easy to fall into a guilt trap after emotional eating, berating yourself for the occasional splurge or slip-up. However, practicing self-kindness is crucial. Instead of dwelling on moments of perceived failure, embrace them as opportunities to learn more about yourself and your needs. Intuitive eating, which emphasizes listening to your body's hunger signals over external cues, can also play a significant role. You nurture a more harmonious relationship with food by tuning into what your body genuinely craves physically and emotionally.

Building resilience against emotional eating involves strengthening your emotional intelligence. This means becoming more aware of how emotions affect your decisions and learning to manage them effectively. When we enhance our emotional understanding, we reduce the tendency to seek solace in food. Social connections play a pivotal role here; they offer support systems that provide comfort and empathy, reducing the need to turn to food for emotional fulfillment. Regular mindfulness practices can further bolster this resilience, promoting a balanced mind that finds peace beyond the dinner table.

Cultivating an environment that supports mindful eating also adds a layer of reinforcement against emotional eating. These small changes foster mindful eating practices, whether it's creating a calming space for meals, setting meal times free from distractions, or encouraging shared family dinners that focus on connection rather than consumption. When everyone in the household aligns with such values, it creates an atmosphere where healthy eating behaviors flourish naturally, making emotional eating less likely to take center stage.

Core Message

Navigating the chaotic realm of mindful eating amid modern life's rapid pace requires grasping its inherent challenges and understanding the subtle yet powerful influences that sway our food choices. These hurdles can seem daunting, from the pressure of fast-paced schedules pushing us towards convenient options to the seemingly innocent distractions of multitasking meals. Yet, the power to shift isn't elusive. We can carve out moments of peace and connection with our food by creating mindful eating rituals, whether dedicating undisturbed meal time or fostering supportive workplace environments. Moreover, understanding the tricks of food marketing and maintaining awareness in bustling convenience stores allows us to reclaim control, choosing nourishment over quick fixes.

In tandem with these behavioral shifts, addressing emotional eating is vital. Recognizing and understanding emotional triggers, like stress or boredom, empowers us to respond with empathy rather than impulsivity. Embracing mindfulness practices and self-compassion nurtures a healthier relationship with food. Building resilience through emotional intelligence equips us to manage feelings better, preventing food from becoming a substitute for emotional fulfillment. Cultivating a support system and sharing meals free of distractions enhances this journey. Creating environments conducive to mindful eating further aligns our actions with intention, allowing us to savor each bite and embrace the joy of eating with clarity and purpose.

"The most important time in life is
always the present."

Mitsuo Aida

Chapter 7

Cultivating Body Awareness

Cultivating body awareness is about tuning into those subtle signals your body sends, especially regarding hunger. Imagine discerning if that gnawing feeling in your stomach is a genuine call for nourishment or just an emotional echo of the day's stresses. Many people go through life disconnected from these signals, often confusing emotional urges with genuine hunger cues. This inattentiveness can lead to unhealthy eating patterns and an overall disconnection from one's physical needs. By fostering a deeper connection with our body's messages, we open avenues for healthier choices that align with our nutritional needs rather than reactive desires.

In this chapter, we will navigate various practices designed to enhance your body awareness, focusing mainly on how they pertain to recognizing hunger signals. You'll explore techniques like using a hunger scale to determine what your body truly craves and employing mindful meal scheduling that respects your natural rhythms. We'll delve into the benefits of maintaining a hunger journal to uncover patterns that might go unnoticed. Additionally, you'll learn to differentiate between emotional cravings and physical hunger through self-inquiry and reflection. Discover how thoughtful practices such as the body scan and meditative eating can further hone your ability to tune into bodily sensations. Each approach serves as a tool to facilitate a more mindful, intentional relationship with food, transforming every meal into an opportunity for nourishment not just for the body but also for the mind.

Practices for Tuning into Natural Hunger Cues

Understanding how to interpret your body's hunger signals is valuable in the journey toward mindful eating. It's about distinguishing between signs of physical hunger and the sudden urges driven by emotions. Often, we mistake stress or boredom for hunger, leading to unnecessary eating and less healthful dietary choices. Instead, learning to listen to our bodies allows us to make better decisions about what, when, and how much to eat.

One effective method is using a hunger scale, which can be incredibly enlightening. Think of a simple scale from one to ten, where one indicates a state of extreme hunger and ten represents feeling uncomfortably full. Applying this scale before meals helps you assess whether you're genuinely hungry or whether other factors are at play. For instance, if you find yourself at a five, you might decide whether to wait a little longer until you genuinely need food or choose a light snack that satisfies without leading to overeating.

Taking this approach a step further involves being mindful about your meal scheduling. Instead of rigid meal times dictated by clocks or social norms, try aligning your eating habits with your body's natural hunger rhythms. This practice can prevent overindulgence fueled by waiting too long to eat, often consuming more significant portions than necessary. By simply listening to your body and respecting its signals, you nurture a balance that contributes to satisfaction and well-being.

Journaling is another powerful practice that supports the cultivation of body awareness. By keeping a diary of your hunger experiences—when you feel hungry, what you eat, and how you feel afterward—you can uncover patterns and triggers associated with your eating habits. Maybe you'll notice that certain situations or emotions consistently lead to craving particular foods. Perhaps you'll recognize that you skip breakfast and overeat at lunch. Writing these experiences down not only aids in understanding but also promotes accountability and reflection on adjusting your habits for the better.

Listening to your body's signals requires a curious and open mindset. It's important to remember that emotional cravings often masquerade as hunger. These cravings might arise from various sources, such as stress, anxiety, or even happiness. To tell them apart, pause and ask yourself questions like: "What am I really feeling?" or "Am I truly hungry?" Over time, this habit of self-inquiry strengthens your ability to make conscious, deliberate decisions about food.

The hunger scale isn't just a tool—it's a guide to self-reflection. It prompts you to explore your internal cues and make more informed choices. Before reaching for that bag of chips or slice of cake, consider where you stand on the scale. Are you indeed famished, or could a glass of water suffice? These small evaluations accumulate into greater awareness and self-control over time.

Mindful meal scheduling emphasizes tuning into your body's needs rather than adhering strictly to traditional meal times. While societal norms suggest three square meals a day, many people find themselves grazing throughout the day or skipping meals due to busy schedules. By observing when you naturally feel hungry and planning meals accordingly, you can maintain energy levels and avoid the pitfalls of getting too hungry, which tends to result in impulsive eating.

Journaling your hunger experiences facilitates more profound insights into your eating patterns. It's not merely about tracking food intake; it's about documenting the thoughts, feelings, and circumstances that influence your eating behavior. As you lay these observations out, patterns begin to emerge. You might discover, for example, that late-night snacking is linked to watching television or that stressful workdays lead to increased caffeine and sugar consumption. Uncovering these links empowers you to implement changes that align with your health goals.

These practices collectively work to heighten your senses and connection to your body. They encourage a shift from mindless to mindful eating—transforming food consumption into an intentional act rather than a reactionary one. Each meal becomes an opportunity to nourish the body and mind, bringing satisfaction and pleasure into eating.

Mind-Body Connection Enhancement Techniques

In today's fast-paced world, many of us have lost the ability to listen to our bodies' natural signals. Fortunately, cultivating body awareness can help us reconnect with these crucial cues, particularly when recognizing hunger. Enhancing the mind-body connection becomes essential.

To begin this journey, incorporating breathing exercises before meals can create a calm and receptive state, allowing us to be better attuned to our hunger signals. Imagine sitting down at the dining table after a long day. Instead of diving straight into your meal, take a moment to close your eyes and inhale deeply through your nose, filling your chest and abdomen. Hold for a few seconds, then slowly exhale through your mouth. Repeat this several times. This simple practice encourages relaxation, reduces stress, and opens the gateway to more mindful eating.

Guidelines for practicing practical breathing exercises include setting aside five minutes before meals to focus on these deep breaths, ensuring a distraction-free environment by turning off electronic devices, and perhaps even dimming the lights or lighting a candle to promote tranquility further. Over time, this routine foster peace and empowers you to detect whether you're starving or eating out of habit or emotion.

Another invaluable tool in connecting with our bodily needs is the body scan. This mindfulness meditation exercise sharpens our attunement to physical sensations related to eating. Picture yourself lying comfortably on your back, eyes gently closed. Start by directing your focus onto your toes, noticing any feelings of warmth, coolness, tension, or relaxation. Slowly work your way up through each part of your body: feet, legs, torso, arms, and finally your head. This exploration increases body awareness, helping distinguish between actual hunger and other sensations that might masquerade as hunger, such as boredom or anxiety.

When performing a body scan, it's crucial to approach it with an open, nonjudgmental mindset. Trust whatever sensations arise without trying to change them. If you're new to this practice, use guided recordings; they can provide structure and support as you become more familiar with the process. Consistency plays a key role here—integrating the body scan into your routine, perhaps once or twice a week, yields the most benefits.

Movement and awareness practices like yoga also enhance the detection of hunger signals through heightened bodily awareness. Yoga, with its emphasis on connecting breath and movement, invites practitioners to explore their physical boundaries while maintaining a conscious presence. Whether it's a gentle Hatha class or a more vigorous Vinyasa flow, yoga teaches us to pay close attention to how our bodies feel in different postures and transitions. This translates into a deeper understanding of hunger cues as we grow more accustomed to listening to and interpreting our body's signals during and after a session.

Those interested in integrating yoga into their lives should start with a beginner's class or online session. Opt for classes emphasizing mindfulness and internal focus rather than purely fitness-driven goals. Remember that consistency is more beneficial than intensity; even brief daily sessions of 15–20 minutes can substantially enhance your bodily awareness over time.

Lastly, meditative eating can establish pre-meal mindfulness, promoting reflection on food gratitude and intentions. Before consuming your meal, take a moment to sincerely appreciate your food's journey to your plate. Consider the elements—sun, rain, soil—that have contributed to its growth, the hands that harvested it, and the love with which it was prepared. Reflecting on these facets sets the stage for an intentional eating experience, where each bite is savored and its nourishment acknowledged.

Approaching meals with gratitude does more than deepen appreciation for the food; it encourages a focused and present mindset during consumption. Take small bites, chew slowly, and engage fully with the flavor and texture of each morsel. Pay attention to how your body reacts as you eat—is there an immediate sense of satisfaction, or are there still lingering sensations of hunger? Such awareness enhances your meal's enjoyment and provides valuable insights into your body's needs and responses.

Building a Routine around Body Checks

Establishing regular routines for assessing hunger and physical states can significantly impact one's health journey. The idea is to create moments that allow us to pause and consider our body's signals, enhancing mindfulness in eating habits and overall well-being. One practical approach is implementing scheduled body checks. Setting aside specific times each day to check in with your body helps cultivate a habit of reflection. These moments can tie into natural breaks in the day, such as mid-morning or mid-afternoon, when energy levels fluctuate. By routinely asking yourself how hungry you feel, what your energy level is like, and if there are any physical signs of hunger, you can begin to recognize patterns in how your body communicates its needs.

Moreover, integrating these checks into your daily tasks reinforces them as natural parts of your routine. Think about pairing body awareness with activities you do every day, like brushing your teeth or taking a shower. Such integration ensures that tuning into your body becomes as regular as these daily rituals, making it easier to maintain over time. For example, take a moment to assess your physical state while preparing your morning coffee or tea. Are you genuinely hungry, or are other factors influencing your desire to eat? Small, consistent practices in your daily routine strengthen your awareness and responsiveness to accurate hunger cues.

Creating a supportive environment also plays a crucial role in enhancing body awareness. Mindfulness begins at home, particularly in spaces where meal preparation takes place. A clutter-free, organized kitchen encourages thoughtful eating habits. By arranging your cooking and dining areas to be calm and inviting, you promote positive food experiences. This could mean keeping healthy snacks visible and storing less healthy options out of immediate sight, thus fostering an environment conducive to mindful eating. Creating a mindset that values nutrition and sustenance can profoundly influence how you interact with food.

Community check-ins should be considered. Engaging with others on similar journeys fosters shared experiences and accountability. By participating in group discussions about body awareness, you gain valuable insights from diverse perspectives, which can deepen your understanding and commitment to mindful eating. Whether through online forums, local meetups, or support groups, finding a community can provide encouragement and validation, making cultivating body awareness more enriching and sustainable. These interactions can generate new ideas and strategies for better connecting with your body's signals and help hold you accountable to your routines.

Final Insights

Understanding and connecting with your body's hunger signals is vital to nurturing mindful eating habits. This chapter explored various practices to help you recognize these signals more clearly. From using a hunger scale to journaling experiences, each method encourages a deeper awareness of what your body truly needs. By integrating mindfulness into meal scheduling and confronting emotional cravings, you can make food choices that satisfy both body and soul. These strategies allow for a more intentional approach to eating, where every bite contributes positively to your health journey.

Enhancing the mind-body connection further supports this mindful eating process. Whether through breathing exercises before meals, engaging in yoga, or practicing body scans, these techniques foster greater bodily awareness and discernment of accurate hunger cues. Building routines around regular body checks helps solidify these practices as everyday habits, creating a supportive environment conducive to thoughtful food interactions. By fostering community connections and maintaining an organized kitchen, the path towards mindful eating becomes enriched with shared knowledge and personal accountability. Embrace this journey with curiosity and patience, knowing each step brings you closer to a healthier, more satisfying relationship with food.

93

"Gratitude turns what we have into enough."

Anonymous.

Chapter 8

Enhancing Gratitude Towards Food

Enhancing gratitude towards food is about much more than simply recognizing it as a source of sustenance. It encourages us to delve into the deeper dimensions of our relationship with what we eat, connecting us to the broader ecosystem and human efforts in food production. It's easy to overlook these connections in our busy lives as we rush through meals. Yet, pausing allows us to acknowledge the intricate network that brings food to our tables, from the nourishing sun and rain to the diligent hands of farmers and workers across the supply chain.

This chapter explores various practices that can transform how we perceive and engage with food. We'll discuss mindful reflection as a tool for appreciating the journey of each meal, emphasizing how it leads us to recognize the contributions of nature and humanity. Simple verbal expressions of gratitude and the creation of personal rituals can foster an environment of appreciation, enriching both our dining experiences and relationships. Furthermore, maintaining a gratitude journal offers a reflective space to deepen awareness and embed thankfulness into everyday life. By engaging in these practices, we cultivate a gratitude mindset beyond eating, fostering a harmonious balance between body and mind. Ultimately, this chapter invites readers to integrate these mindful practices into their routines, promoting a culture of gratitude that enhances emotional well-being and supports sustainable living.

Gratitude Practices Before Meals

Cultivating a mindset of gratitude before eating can be a transformative practice that enriches our emotional health and enhances how we nourish our bodies. In our fast-paced lives, meal times often become rushed moments we push through rather than cherish. However, by slowing down and practicing mindful reflection, we can begin to appreciate the intricate contributions involved in bringing food to our table.

Mindful reflection invites us to pause, breathe, and acknowledge the immense network of nature and human effort behind every bite. Consider the sun's nurturing rays, the soil's rich nutrients, and the rain's gentle nourishment—all vital elements in the growth of the plants and animals that provide sustenance. Then, add the hard work of farmers, the hands of harvesters, drivers transporting goods, and retailers stocking shelves. Each step is a reminder of interdependence, a testament to the collaborative dance between humanity and nature. To practice this, take a moment before meals to consciously reflect on these processes. Visualize the journey of your food, from earth to plate, and allow gratitude to well up for each link in this chain.

Simple expressions of gratitude can be powerful complements to mindful reflection. Before diving into your meal, consider expressing a sentence or two of thanks. These verbal acknowledgments need not be elaborate—a heartfelt "Thank you" directed towards your food, the people who prepared it, or the universe that provides it can create a meaningful shift in perspective. This small gesture cultivates a positive atmosphere, enriching the dining experience and setting the tone for mindful consumption.

Furthermore, creating personal or family rituals around meal times can reinforce expressing gratitude as a consistent practice. Rituals don't have to be complex; they might involve lighting a candle, playing calming music, or sharing what you are thankful for with your dining companions. By doing so, you establish an environment where gratitude is naturally woven into the fabric of everyday life. Sharing these moments fosters connections among family members, making meal times more than just about food but also about togetherness and appreciation for one another and the world.

Encouraging the keeping of a gratitude journal focused on meals and food experiences is another profound way to deepen this practice. Journaling provides a reflective space to explore your relationship with food further. As you jot down daily reflections, consider noting what you enjoyed about the meal, any new flavors you experienced, memories invoked, or thoughts on the sources of your ingredients. This exercise promotes mindfulness, allowing you to savor the sensory experience of eating while embedding gratitude into your consciousness.

To start maintaining a gratitude journal, choose a suitable time, such as a few minutes after dinner, to unwind and reflect. Document specific instances, like enjoying a fresh berry pie made with summer fruits or appreciating the comfort of a warm meal on a cold day. Over time, you'll likely notice a heightened sense of awareness around food and its role in your life, bridging the connection between emotional well-being and physical nourishment.

By engaging in mindful reflection, verbal gratitude, developing rituals, and journaling, we gradually cultivate a deeper appreciation for food that transcends mere sustenance. This approach animates our relationship with what we eat and enhances our overall well-being. Embracing gratitude in this manner enriches our emotional landscape, promoting a harmonious balance between body and mind. Recognizing the interconnected forces that sustain us elevates eating from a basic necessity to a cherished ritual, fostering physical and emotional nourishment.

Emphasizing a gratitude-focused mindset creates rippling effects that extend beyond individual benefits. Communities built on a shared appreciation for food nurture a culture of mindfulness, compassion, and empathy. This collective understanding strengthens bonds, encourages sustainable practices, and fosters a healthier relationship with our environment. While the hustle of modern life can make such pauses challenging, the rewards are immeasurable, impacting how we perceive and interact with the world.

Understanding the Journey of Food to Plate

In our daily lives, it's easy to take the food on our plates for granted, yet each meal represents a complex journey that deserves recognition. To genuinely appreciate food availability, we must first increase awareness of the intricate processes from production to consumption. By delving into this journey, we develop an appreciation beyond mere sustenance.

First, let's explore the stages of food production. Beginning with farming, it's essential to recognize the dedication and hard work farmers invest in nurturing crops or raising livestock. Farmers spend long hours ensuring their produce's health and growth, dealing with weather conditions, pests, and soil quality. For instance, growing wheat involves numerous steps: preparing the land, planting seeds, monitoring plant health, and harvesting at the right time. All these stages require knowledge, patience, and skill, which we often overlook when enjoying a slice of bread.

After the initial farming comes the process of harvesting. This step varies depending on the crop or animal product type but always demands precision and care. Whether picking ripe fruits by hand or using machinery for large-scale grain collection, harvesting celebrates the efforts invested throughout the season. It marks the transition from the farm to the next stage: processing.

Processing transforms raw ingredients into consumable goods. It ranges from simple activities, like washing and packaging, to more complex procedures, such as milling grains into flour or fermenting grapes into wine. Each method adds value and accessibility to the original product while ensuring its safety and longevity. Consider milk; once collected, it's pasteurized and homogenized, making it safe and palatable.

Understanding these transformations invites us to appreciate the multitude of hands and technologies contributing to our everyday meals.

Examining cultural perspectives provides deeper insight into how different societies respect and honor their food origins. In Japan, "itadakimasu" before meals is a form of gratitude, acknowledging the life forms sacrificed and the people who worked hard to bring the food to the table. Similarly, Indigenous communities might perform rituals or dances celebrating their harvests, showing reverence for nature's gifts.

Such cultural practices underscore the importance of understanding food and identity. Cuisine, imbued with history and tradition, shapes cultural identities. For example, the Indigenous Hawaiian practice of "luau" serves as a communal feast and a testament to their respect for the land and seas that provide sustenance. Learning about these traditions encourages us to reevaluate our food customs and consider integrating meaningful practices into our daily routines.

Another significant factor impacting our appreciation for food is understanding its environmental footprint. Our choices have far-reaching effects on ecosystems across the globe. Selecting sustainably sourced products promotes healthier environments and ensures future food security. Opting for organic vegetables supports soil health, diminishes chemical exposure, and encourages biodiversity. Furthermore, reducing meat consumption lessens greenhouse gas emissions, alleviating climate change pressures. These small shifts in our consumer habits can generate substantial positive outcomes for the planet.

Thus, sustainable practices should be seen as a responsibility rather than a trend. Being informed about where our food comes from, how it was produced, and the implications of our dietary decisions empowers us to make conscious choices. For instance, supporting local farmers' markets reduces transportation emissions and contributes to local economies. When we understand the broader impacts of our consumption patterns, we enhance our connection to the world around us and cultivate gratitude for our resources.

Finally, incorporating rituals during food preparation can further deepen our connection to its journey. We cultivate mindfulness and appreciation by acknowledging the origins and effort behind our ingredients. Simple practices such as taking a moment to express gratitude before cooking or discussing the source of ingredients with family members can transform routine meals into opportunities for reflection. One might light a candle or play music that resonates with the cultural heritage of the prepared dish, enhancing the dining experience with intentionality and respect.

When we consciously integrate these rituals, we weave thankfulness into the fabric of our culinary practices. Cooking becomes not merely a necessity but a celebration of life's abundance. Through this lens of gratitude, we elevate our relationship with food beyond physical nourishment, fostering a holistic connection that nourishes both body and soul.

Cultural Rituals Involving Food Contemplation

In many cultures, traditional practices surrounding food are deeply rooted in expressions of gratitude and mindfulness. These practices often begin with blessings before meals, serving as a moment to thank the earth for its bounty and acknowledge the hard work that brought the food to the table. In India, for example, it is common for families to express gratitude through prayers or mantras, which offer thanks while promoting mindfulness about the meal's significance. Similarly, some Japanese customs involve the phrase "Itadakimasu," which reflects humility and appreciation for those who cultivated and prepared the food.

These rituals are not limited to religious contexts but extend into everyday life across different societies. They encourage individuals to pause, reflect, and connect emotionally with the sustenance provided. By incorporating these small acts into daily routines, individuals can cultivate an ongoing awareness of food's value beyond physical nourishment.

Moving from individual practices to communal settings, many cultures utilize shared meals to foster relationships and deepen gratitude. The concept of sharing food resonates universally, and gatherings like the Italian "Festa di San Giovanni" or the American Thanksgiving are prime examples of communal eating transcending ordinary dining experiences. These events provide opportunities for communities to come together, reinforcing bonds and expressing appreciation for one another's company.

Guidelines for hosting communal meals emphasize inclusivity and understanding. Encouraging diverse contributions from participants allows everyone to bring a piece of their heritage to the table. This practice enhances the variety of dishes and promotes cultural exchange and mutual respect. Including everyone in meal preparations and discussions around the table helps underscore the communal aspect of dining, reminding participants that food is as much about human connection as it is about sustenance.

Embracing cultural practices that encourage savoring each bite can enhance the food experience. The French tradition of "joie de vivre" highlights the pleasure of enjoying life's simple moments, including eating. This mindset encourages individuals to take their time during meals, appreciating intricate flavors and textures. Such practices discourage rushing through meals and promote a more deliberate, mindful approach to eating.

Mindful eating guidelines suggest focusing on sensory experiences—observing colors, inhaling aromas, tasting nuances, and feeling textures. Engaging fully with these senses can transform eating into a meditative act, grounding individuals in the present moment while deepening their appreciation for the meal. Practicing this regularly can help shift focus from quantity to quality, encouraging healthier dietary habits and a more profound sense of gratitude.

Ceremonies and rituals surrounding food are pivotal in marking critical transitions or celebrations within various cultures. The Chinese Lantern Festival is one such ceremony that symbolizes family unity and prosperity, celebrated with an array of foods believed to bring good luck. In indigenous cultures across North America, potlatch ceremonies are significant social and economic events, emphasizing gift-giving and reciprocity associated with shared feasts.

While these ceremonies are rich in cultural history, they also provide guidelines for integrating meaningful traditions into modern contexts. Participating in or adapting these rituals can imbue regular meals with a greater sense of purpose and collective memory. Individuals might consider introducing elements of such ceremonies into their own lives, using them as opportunities to honor personal milestones or gather loved ones in celebration.

Final Thoughts

This chapter explored how cultivating gratitude practices before meals can transform our food experience. By slowing down and mindfully reflecting on the journey from earth to plate, we gain a deeper appreciation for the intricate processes and efforts involved. Simple acts, such as expressing thanks or creating personal rituals, enhance our emotional connection with meal times. These practices encourage an appreciation for food beyond mere sustenance and foster togetherness and mindfulness in our daily lives. Journaling about food experiences further enriches this mindset, allowing us to savor flavors and moments while embedding gratitude into our consciousness.

Our appreciation extends beyond individual benefits as we understand food's journey and cultural significance. Embracing sustainable choices reinforces our responsibility towards the environment and fosters healthier relationships with our surroundings. Rituals and mindful eating create a holistic connection that nourishes both body and soul, transforming meals into cherished moments of celebration and reflection. Through these approaches, we nurture communities built on shared appreciation, empathy, and understanding, ultimately enriching our overall well-being and connection to the world.

"The purpose of life is a life of purpose."

Robert Byrne

Chapter 9

Lessons from Okinawan Elders

Exploring the lessons from Okinawan elders offers a glimpse into the vibrant tapestry of wisdom and tradition that underpins their prosperous lives. Known for their remarkable longevity, these centenarians are not simply anomalies but are living testaments to lifestyles rich in cultural practices and communal values. Their lives are deeply interwoven with family and community, illustrating how these relationships foster a holistic environment conducive to well-being. Each shared meal and story passed down through generations demonstrates an intrinsic understanding of health as a collective endeavor rather than an individual pursuit. This chapter delves into these aspects, revealing how intergenerational bonds and community participation play pivotal roles in sustaining body and spirit.

Readers will venture into the heart of Okinawan life, where everyday activities seamlessly blend into practices promoting health and harmony. The chapter unveils the vital significance of family dynamics, showing how meal preparation becomes a unifying act that transcends simple nutritional value to embrace cultural continuity and togetherness. It highlights storytelling's profound impact during these gatherings, serving as a method for preserving traditions and as a conduit for imparting crucial life lessons across generations. Furthermore, the narrative explores the extended community's influence on personal health, detailing the social engagements that enhance emotional wellness and foster belonging. By examining the role of older role models, the text presents an enlightening perspective on how traditional practices reinforce modernity without losing essence—ultimately guiding younger generations toward fulfilling lives anchored in timeless virtues.

The Role of Family and Community in Healthy Living

Okinawan elders demonstrate the significant role of intergenerational knowledge and social connections in promoting health and well-being. Central to this is family members sharing responsibilities in meal preparation, reinforcing healthy nutritional habits, and nurturing a sense of community within families. In Okinawa, preparing meals is viewed as a collective activity where every member, from grandchildren to grandparents, contributes. This tradition ensures that everyone is engaged in choosing and preparing fresh, healthy ingredients, thus reinforcing mindful eating as a core value. By participating in meal preparation, younger generations learn the importance of nutrition from their elders, who have accumulated wisdom over decades about what constitutes a balanced diet.

Storytelling during meals is another vital tradition among Okinawan families, serving to pass down cultural traditions and life lessons. This ritual fosters a strong family bond, creating an environment where wisdom flows naturally from one generation to the next. As elders narrate stories of their past experiences and teachings, they provide invaluable life lessons to the younger family members. Stories of resilience, hope, and perseverance become tools for children and grandchildren, equipping them with insights into overcoming challenges. Moreover, this storytelling tradition helps preserve the unique cultural identity of the Okinawan people, ensuring that their rich heritage remains vibrant across generations.

Active participation in community events further highlights the role of social connections in promoting health. In Okinawa, community gatherings are standard, allowing individuals to engage with others outside their immediate family circle. These events often include festivals, group activities, and communal exercise sessions to encourage participant interaction and camaraderie. Such active involvement strengthens social support networks, offering emotional sustenance crucial for mental health. Engaging in communal activities has enhanced overall well-being by providing a sense of belonging and purpose, effectively combating feelings of loneliness and isolation.

Elders in Okinawa stand as role models for younger generations, exemplifying how traditional practices can contribute to overall well-being. By observing their elders, young Okinawans gain firsthand insights into balancing modern life with time-tested customs. The elders' adherence to practices like maintaining an active lifestyle, respecting nature, and prioritizing community over individualism instills valuable lessons in the youth. For instance, regular participation in traditional arts or cooperative work helps young people appreciate the benefits of collaboration and mutual support—a philosophy deeply embedded in Okinawan culture.

Although discussed later in the chapter, physical activity is inherently linked to these social connections. In Okinawa, engaging in physical activities such as gardening or joining neighborhood walking groups is a natural part of life; it's a shared experience that strengthens body and community ties. Notably, while exploring these ideas, it becomes clear that guidelines for seamlessly integrating physical activity into daily routines mirror those foundational intergenerational and social principles, underscoring the harmonious relationship between physical health and social engagement.

The synergy between these elements—family security through shared responsibilities, cultural preservation via storytelling, enhanced well-being through community participation, and direction offered by older role models—forms the bedrock of health promotion in Okinawa. Family meals become more than just sustenance; they evolve into celebrations of culture and generational continuity. Community events cease to be mere gatherings, transforming into essential frameworks for social cohesion and psychological stability. Through these interactions, the young observe and absorb the virtues reflected in their elders' way of life, learning to cherish values that promote a long, fulfilling existence.

Lifestyle Patterns and Philosophies Contributing to Longevity

Okinawan centenarians offer a rich tableau of daily habits and philosophies that contribute significantly to their longevity, beginning with their approach to physical activity. Rather than setting aside dedicated times for exercise, these elders seamlessly incorporate movement into their daily routines through gardening and walking. Gardening is therapeutic and ensures they are on their feet, stretching, bending, and moving naturally. There's no need for gym memberships or structured workout sessions; instead, the rhythm of daily life provides all the exercise they require. Walking to market, tilling the soil, or tending to household chores keeps them physically active in a way that feels less like exercise and more like living.

These effortless integrations of physical activity illustrate the importance of organically embedding exercise into one's lifestyle. When physical exertion is a byproduct of daily tasks rather than a separate obligation, it becomes sustainable and enjoyable. This natural engagement in exercise is contrasted starkly with modern society's often rigid fitness regimens, which can feel burdensome or inaccessible for some. The lesson here is clear: finding joy in daily movement supports both physical health and mental well-being without the pressure of hitting milestones or achieving specific fitness outcomes.

Another cornerstone of Okinawan longevity is the philosophy known as 'Ikigai,' which translates to "a reason for being." This concept emphasizes the importance of having a purpose in life—a driving force that motivates individuals to get up each morning with intention and enthusiasm. Ikigai is intensely personal; it could be a hobby, a professional pursuit, or simply the love of spending time with family. Identifying and nurturing one's ikigai leads to greater fulfillment and healthier lifestyle choices. Studies have shown that having a sense of purpose is linked to improved health outcomes, including reduced risk of cardiovascular disease and depression among older adults.

Cultivating ikigai involves introspection and understanding what truly matters to an individual. To embark on this path, consider what activities light you up, what contributions you wish to make, and how these can be integrated into your daily life. This heartfelt alignment with personal values encourages individuals to prioritize wellness holistically, ultimately improving their quality of life.

A critical aspect of Okinawan dietary habits is rooted in moderation. They practice what's known as "Hara Hachi Bu," roughly meaning "eat until you are 80% full." This discipline reflects restraint and an appreciation of food as a source of joy. Smaller, moderate portions enhance flavor experiences, allowing individuals to savor every bite. This mindful eating approach emphasizes quality over quantity, ensuring that meals are satisfying and nourishing.

This practice challenges modern notions of consumption, where portion sizes are often exaggerated, leading to overindulgence. Individuals can improve their relationship with food by adopting a similar attitude toward eating, focusing on moderation, and celebrating food as a joyful experience. It's not merely about sustenance; it's about cherishing the flavors and nourishing oneself, which contributes positively to physical health and emotional well-being.

The resilience and adaptability of Okinawan elders are evident through their personal stories of overcoming adversity. Their lives are testaments to enduring change while holding onto essential cultural practices. Many have lived through significant historical events and societal changes yet exhibit remarkable adaptability. By integrating new ideas and technologies into their lives when advantageous, they demonstrate openness while remaining grounded in traditions that support their well-being.

Embracing change allows these centenarians to stay relevant and engaged with the world around them. It's a mindset that welcomes progress but does not discard valuable cultural heritage. For anyone seeking longevity and fulfillment, learning to balance these dynamics—openness to change with reverence for tradition—is a helpful guideline. Change is inevitable, but how we respond can significantly shape our experiences and outcomes.

Final Thoughts

Okinawan centenarians demonstrate how intertwined family, traditions, and community are with prolonged life and well-being. This chapter has highlighted the unique ways these elements interconnect, from shared meal preparations that promote nutritional learning and familial bonds to the storytelling that transfers cultural wisdom across generations. These practices foster a deep sense of belonging and identity, serving as vital mechanisms for health and happiness. Additionally, participation in community events strengthens social support and combats isolation, effectively enhancing mental and emotional wellness among Okinawans. Young Okinawans learn invaluable lessons in balancing new world challenges with time-honored traditions through observing and emulating their elders.

Moreover, the lifestyle philosophies of Okinawans, such as integrating physical activity naturally into daily routines and adhering to the principles of ikigai and Hara Hachi Bu, offer essential insights into sustaining healthful living. They maintain physical vitality without additional stress by viewing exercise as part of life rather than an obligation. Their commitment to purposeful living encourages healthier choices, while mindful eating underscores the joy and moderation in consumption. The adaptability and resilience of these elders, even in the face of change, further illustrate the importance of merging beneficial innovations with traditional values. Together, these elements underscore a holistic approach to longevity, offering valuable guidance for anyone seeking a fulfilling and balanced life.

118

"He who strongly desires to rise will
think of a way to build a ladder."

Japanese proverb

Chapter 10

Starting Your Journey: A Holistic Approach

Embarking on a balanced and mindful eating journey is like setting sail on a personal adventure toward well-being. It's a path that invites you to befriend your body's needs while nurturing a sustainable approach to food that fuels both body and soul. This chapter delves into the art of creating a personalized plan for mindful eating, urging you to embrace strategies that harmonize with your lifestyle. From setting pragmatic goals to navigating the landscape of emotional eating triggers, we introduce techniques to foster lasting positive change without overwhelming rigidity. As you turn each page, you'll uncover insights designed to transform your relationship with food, moving beyond the constraints of diet culture into a practice of thoughtful nourishment.

In this chapter, you will discover how to tailor your mindful eating journey to suit your unique circumstances. We explore the importance of establishing SMART goals and how these objectives can guide your path to healthier habits. Learn about the power of meal planning and how organizing your living space supports your intentions by minimizing temptation. The chapter also illuminates the role of emotions in shaping eating behaviors and offers practical tools to manage them beyond reaching for comfort food. By integrating diverse foods and practicing self-compassion in times of setbacks, you'll cultivate an environment conducive to sustainable eating habits. Prepare to embark on a holistic expedition where dietary choices are more than mere actions—they become affirmations of a vibrant, balanced life.

Creating a Personal Action Plan

When starting your journey toward mindful eating, developing a personalized strategy that fits your unique lifestyle is essential. This journey begins by setting SMART goals—specific, measurable, achievable, relevant, and time-bound objectives. By defining clear targets, such as replacing processed foods with whole, organic produce over the next month, you create a clear path forward. This clarity helps you maintain focus and commitment.

Additionally, SMART goals are not fixed; they are adaptable. You can revise them as you progress to align with your changing challenges and achievements. This flexibility is crucial in a world where life often doesn't go as planned.

Next, planning your meals can significantly help prevent impulsive eating. It encourages you to make conscious choices rather than grabbing whatever is readily available when hunger strikes. One principle to consider is Hara Hachi Bu, a Japanese concept that advises eating until you are 80% full. This principle emphasizes portion control and mindfulness during meals, helping you prioritize nutrition over convenience.

Preparing meals in advance also allows you to include a variety of nutrients and flavors. This approach makes it easier to stick to healthier options without feeling deprived.

Creating a supportive home environment can help you eat mindfully. Start by changing your living space to remove temptations. Please eliminate unhealthy snacks and processed foods to reduce the chances of eating them without thinking. Instead, fill your kitchen with healthy foods that are good for your body and mind, like fresh fruits, vegetables, nuts, and whole grains. An organized kitchen or pantry shows your commitment to healthy choices and supports your eating efforts.

Monitoring your progress is an essential part of a comprehensive approach to wellness. Utilize journals or apps to record your dietary selections, emotional triggers, and eating habits. By tracking your consumption and subsequent feelings, you can pinpoint which foods promote your well-being and which might hinder it. For instance, you may discover that certain dishes leave you feeling revitalized and alert while others result in fatigue or discomfort. With this insight, you can make well-informed changes to your eating plan, ensuring it caters to your needs effectively.

Reflect on how emotions influence eating habits. Many people turn to food for comfort during stress or emotional upheaval, often leading to overeating or poor food choices. Keeping a journal helps track what you eat and how you feel before and after meals. Noticing patterns between emotional states and eating habits enables you to strategize better ways to cope with emotions beyond using food as a crutch. Engaging in a short walk or practicing breathing exercises could become alternative responses to stress, aligned with your mindful eating goals.

Additionally, consider introducing new tools and techniques gradually. If you're using an app to monitor your intake, try integrating features that allow for measuring macronutrient distribution or hydration levels, but do so one step at a time. Overloading yourself with too many changes at once can overwhelm you, whereas incremental adoption ensures each new habit has time to take root.

Maintaining Long-Term Commitment without Rigidity

Flexibility is crucial to sustaining a mindful eating practice over time. It's easy to view nutritional guidelines as rigid rules, but life doesn't operate under such strict parameters. Embracing adaptability means recognizing that life's changes are inevitable and that an inflexible approach to eating might only sometimes be feasible. Allowing indulgences without guilt promotes resilience and cultivates a healthier relationship with food.

Consider the scenario where you plan to eat healthily for a week, but you're invited to a celebration filled with delicious treats halfway through. Instead of feeling guilty about enjoying these delights, adaptability encourages you to accept the moment as a part of life's richness. It helps you realize that consistent effort is more beneficial than striving for perfection in every meal. This shift in mindset nurtures a more forgiving and balanced approach to dietary habits.

Incorporating flexibility into your eating habits also ties into setting realistic expectations. Setting goals that align with your lifestyle, including small and significant milestones, is essential. By breaking down larger objectives into incremental steps, you prevent burnout. For instance, incorporate one meat-free meal weekly to transition to a plant-based diet. As you grow comfortable with each step, gradually increase your commitment. Each milestone becomes an opportunity for celebration, fueling enthusiasm and fostering sustained positive change despite occasional setbacks.

Setting realistic expectations isn't just about achieving long-term goals; it's about cultivating an environment where you regularly acknowledge your progress. Let's say you've decided to reduce sugar intake. Instead of eliminating all sugar immediately, you could replace your morning sugary snack with fruit. Celebrate this change, understanding that even seemingly minor adjustments contribute to your well-being. This mindful practice diminishes feelings of overwhelm and keeps the journey enjoyable.

Variety is another critical factor in preventing monotony and making healthy eating sustainable. Introducing diverse, whole foods into your diet opens you to flavors and textures. Exploring new recipes can transform meals from routine to experiences worth relishing. Imagine swapping your usual salad for a vibrant medley of roasted vegetables tossed in olive oil and herbs. Not only does this diversify your palate, it also ensures you get a broader spectrum of nutrients, enhancing overall health.

Diversity in food choices can also stimulate creativity in the kitchen. Trying different cuisines or incorporating seasonal produce into your meals can make cooking an exciting adventure. Perhaps you've never cooked with quinoa before—experimenting with it as a staple ingredient can invigorate your culinary repertoire, keeping meals refreshing rather than predictable. The excitement of trying something new makes it easier to maintain motivation on your journey toward mindful eating.

However, even with the best intentions, setbacks happen. Practicing self-compassion during these times is essential. When you experience a setback, such as overeating at a party, it's vital to reframe negative self-talk into constructive reflections. Rather than dwelling on perceived failures, remind yourself that every meal offers a chance for a fresh start. This perspective shift empowers you to move beyond momentary lapses without derailing your progress.

Cultivating self-compassion requires acknowledging that everyone faces challenges on their health journeys. You might find it helpful to keep a journal where you record your thoughts and emotions surrounding food choices. Doing so gives you insight into patterns that trigger setbacks and develop strategies to navigate them more effectively. Focusing on long-term well-being rather than short-term missteps fosters resilience and a positive outlook.

Bringing It All Together

Finding balance and mindfulness in our eating habits is not just about following rules but creating a lifestyle that feels right for you. This chapter outlined the essentials of developing a personal action plan, starting with SMART goals that allow flexibility as life changes. Planning meals helps you make intelligent choices about what you eat. This way, you can feed your body healthy foods while following ideas like Hara Hachi Bu. Tracking your progress with journals or apps gives you helpful information to adjust your plan for better results. Understanding your feelings about food and finding healthier ways to deal with life's challenges is essential.

As you begin this journey, remember that being adaptable is essential. Life will continually present challenges, so welcoming flexibility can help preserve your motivation and enjoyment in mindful eating habits. Making enduring changes involves establishing realistic, attainable goals that integrate smoothly into your daily life. Whether trying new recipes or slowly shifting to different dietary patterns, variety adds excitement and sustainability. Acknowledge every small success you achieve, even when you face setbacks. By handling these instances with self-kindness and strength, you'll nurture a positive relationship with food, emphasizing progress and optimism rather than perfection.

"If a man has no tea (in him), he is incapable of understanding truth and beauty."

Chapter 11

The Flavors of Okinawa

Okinawa Island stands out for its impressive population of centenarians, a phenomenon linked mainly to its wholesome lifestyle and nutrient-dense traditional diet. Explore the renowned dishes and ingredients from Okinawa that play a crucial role in promoting their remarkable longevity:

1. Goya Champuru (Bitter Melon Stir-Fry)

Key Ingredients:

- Bitter melon (Goya)
- Tofu
- egg
- Pork or fish
- Vegetables

Why It's Healthy:

- Bitter melon rich in antioxidants
- Vitamin C
- Fiber
- Tofu provides plant-based protein and isoflavones suitable for heart health

2. Okinawa Soba

Key Ingredients:

- Wheat noodles
- Pork broth
- Braised pork belly
- Green onions
- Pickled ginger

Why It's Healthy:

- Richer than some dishes
- Eaten sparingly
- Broth contains collagen from pork, which supports skin and joint health

3. Umibudo (Sea Grapes)

Key Ingredients:

- Type of fresh seaweed served as a salad ingredient.

Why It's Healthy:

- High in minerals like iodine and magnesium
- Supports thyroid and bone health
- It contains fucoidan, a compound with anti-inflammatory and anti-cancer properties

4. Tofu Dishes

Key Variants:

- Shima tofu (Island-style Tofu)
- Tofu-soup
- Stir-fried tofu dishes

Why It's Healthy:

- Tofu is a low-calorie
- High-protein food
- Supports muscle maintenance
- Cardiovascular health

5. Mozuku Seaweed Salad

Key Ingredients:

- Mozuku seaweed
- Vinegar
- Soy sauce
- Sesame

Why It's Healthy:

- Packed with polysaccharides
- Boost the immune system
- High in dietary fiber and antioxidants

6. Rafute (Braised Pork Belly)

Key Ingredients:

- Pork belly simmered in soy sauce
- Sugar
- Awamori (Okinawan rice liquor)

Why It's Healthy:

- Fatty
- Consumed in small portions
- Provides collagen and
- Provide energy

7. Purple Sweet Potato (Beni Imo)

How It's Eaten:

- Boiled
- Steamed
- Incorporated into desserts

Why It's Healthy:

- High in antioxidants (anthocyanins),
- Vitamin A
- High in fiber
- Carbohydrate source with a low glycemic index.

8. Mimiga (Pig's Ear Salad)

Key Ingredients:

- Thinly sliced pig's ear
- Vinegar
- Soy sauce
- Vegetables

Why It's Healthy:

- Rich in collagen

- Supports skin
- Supports joint health
- Consumed in small quantities

9. Vegetables and Stir-Fried Greens

Key Ingredients: Local vegetables like Shikuwasa (citrus), carrots, radishes, and mustard greens.

Why It's Healthy:

- High in vitamins
- Fiber
- Phytonutrients
- Lightly stir-fried
- Boiled to preserve nutrients

10. Shikuwasa Citrus

How It's Used:

- As a juice
- Seasoning
- Refreshing drink

Why It's Healthy:

- Rich in vitamin C, flavonoids, and antioxidants
- It supports immune function
- Reduces oxidative stress

11. Turmeric Tea (Ukoncha)

Key Ingredients:

- Ground turmeric
- Hot water

Why It's Healthy:

- Turmeric is anti-inflammatory
- Supports liver health
- Consumed as a daily health tonic.

12. Irabu Soup (Sea Snake Soup)

Key Ingredients:

- Irabu sea snake
- Kelp
- Vegetables

Why It's Healthy:

- High in protein
- Omega-3 fatty acids
- Minerals
- Believed to boost vitality

13. Taimo (Taro Root)

How It's Eaten:

- Boiled
- Mashed
- Used in soups

Why It's Healthy:

- A starchy vegetable
- Rich in complex carbohydrates
- Dietary fiber

14. Fu Champuru (Gluten Stir-Fry)

Key Ingredients:

- Wheat gluten
- Eggs
- Vegetables
- Pork or fish

Why It's Healthy:

- Low in calories
- High in protein
- Combined with nutrient-rich vegetables

15. Black Sugar (Kokuto)

How It's Used:

- Natural sweeteners in teas
- Desserts

Why It's Healthy:

- Unrefined sugar that retains minerals like calcium, potassium, and iron
- It is consumed in moderation

16. Sata Andagi (Okinawan Doughnuts)

Key Ingredients:

- Flour
- Sugar
- Eggs

Why It's Healthy:

- Rare indulgences enjoyed in small portions.

17. Local Fish and Seafood

Common Types:

- Tuna
- mackerel
- squid

Why It's Healthy:

- Rich in omega-3 fatty acids
- Supporting heart
- Brain health

18. Herbs and Spices

Examples:

- Mugwort (Fuchiba),
- turmeric, and
- ginger.

Why It's Healthy:

- These herbs have anti-inflammatory
- Digestive

- Immune-boosting properties

19. Okinawan Rice (Uruchimai)

How It's Eaten:

- Paired with vegetables
- Seaweed
- Fish

Why It's Healthy:

- Low in fat
- Paired with nutrient-dense side dishes

20. Yushi Dofu (Fresh Soft Tofu Soup)

Key Ingredients:

- Silky tofu in a light broth with vegetables

Why It's Healthy:

- High in protein
- Low in fat
- Easy to digest

These dishes and ingredients form Okinawan cuisine's foundation, emphasizing balance, nutrient density, and moderation. Their dietary habits, active lifestyle, and strong community bonds contribute to the remarkable longevity in Okinawa.

Conclusion

Our exploration of Hara Hachi Bu and mindful eating has uncovered essential principles beyond basic dietary habits. At its core, Hara Hachi Bu encourages us to embrace a lifestyle defined by moderation, mindfulness, and respect for tradition. This approach to eating serves not just as a guideline but as an opportunity to cultivate a deeper, more intentional relationship with food—one that can significantly impact our overall well-being.

This text examined the simple yet powerful principle of eating until you are 80% full. This approach encourages us to pause and truly appreciate the act of eating. It's not just about what we put on our plates but also how we engage with each meal, listen to our bodies, and respect our hunger cues. By adopting this practice, we cultivate an awareness beyond the dining table and influence our choices in various aspects of life.

Reflecting on the lessons, consider the benefits of incorporating mindful eating into your daily routine. Imagine dedicating time daily to enjoy a meal, allowing yourself to savor each bite and fully experience the flavors and textures. This practice enhances your awareness and nurtures gratitude for the nourishment that sustains you. Establishing such habits creates a foundation for a healthier and more balanced life.

Better digestion and a sense of fullness that align more closely with your body's nutritional needs can improve your physical health. Perhaps even more significant is the emotional aspect: finding joy in simplicity and satisfaction in moderation can transform your entire perspective on food.

Beyond individual practices, the power of community and support networks cannot be overstated. While embarking on the mindful eating journey might seem solitary at times, connecting with others who share similar goals can anchor your commitment. Imagine joining a local group centered around mindful eating; through sharing experiences and challenges, you contribute to a collective wisdom that enhances everyone's journey. In these communities, accountability meets encouragement, reminding us that we are not alone. Together, you can navigate the complexities of changing habits, celebrate victories—big and small—and find solace in shared understanding.

This cultural practice also invites us to reflect on its origins and the broader themes it represents. By embracing the ethos of Hara Hachi Bu, you engage with a tradition that honors generations of Okinawans who have lived in harmony with their bodies and environments through moderation and mindfulness. There's a profound cultural significance in recognizing how these practices have contributed to health and longevity. By integrating these principles into your modern life, you pay homage to a legacy of wisdom while enriching your experiences. Each mindful meal becomes a bridge between past and present, creating a tapestry of respect for traditions that continue to offer relevance and insight today.

Consider how these lessons extend beyond the realm of eating. Hara Hachi Bu encourages us to apply moderation and mindfulness in all areas of life. Whether we are choosing how to spend our time, managing resources, or setting personal goals, the principles discussed throughout this book guide us toward a balanced existence. This way of living is characterized by intention, where our decisions are based on an understanding of sufficiency rather than excess.

Ultimately, the journey you undertake with Hara Hachi Bu is deeply personal. It invites you to engage more harmoniously with your body and mind, challenging societal norms that often equate abundance with satisfaction. This process is focused on something other than strict rules or unattainable ideals but emphasizes continuous learning and growth. Every mindful choice you make contributes to a larger narrative of change. You take control over your relationship with food, guided by curiosity, compassion, and a sustained commitment.

As you stand on the brink of implementing these insights into your reality, let this conclusion serve as both a reminder and a call to action. Let it reinforce what you've absorbed: mindful eating is an empowering choice that can reshape your approach to food and your outlook on life. With each deliberate bite, you embark on a path toward a harmonious balance, inviting peace, vitality, and fulfillment into your everyday routine.

So, take this wisdom forward, acknowledging the inherent beauty in simplicity and moderation. Understand that this transformation unfolds gradually, one mindful moment at a time. May your journey with Hara Hachi Bu enrich your existence, embodying a life of purpose, awareness, and a profound appreciation for the intricate dance of nourishment and restraint. Here's to the unfolding chapters of your life, inspired by principles that elevate spirit and being.